The American Civil War Surgery Series

Edited by Ira M. Rutkow, M.D., Dr.P.H.

1. S.D. Gross: *A Manual of Military Surgery* (Philadelphia, 1861)

2. S.P. Moore: *A Manual of Military Surgery, Prepared for the Use of the Confederate States Army*. (Richmond, 1863)

3. S.W. Mitchell, G.R. Morehouse and W.W. Keen: *Gunshot Wounds and Other Injuries of Nerves* (Philadelphia, 1864)

4. J.J. Chisolm: *A Manual of Military Surgery* (Richmond, 1861)

5. F.H. Hamilton: *A Practical Treatise on Military Surgery* (New York, 1861)

6. E. Warren: *An Epitome of Practical Surgery for Field and Hospital* (Richmond, 1863)

7. C.S. Tripler and G.C. Blackman: *Handbook for the Military Surgeon* (Cincinnati, 1861)

8. S. Smith: *Hand-book of Surgical Operations* (New York, 1862)

9. F. Formento: *Notes and Observations on Army Surgery* (New Orleans, 1863), bound with:

   M. Schuppert: *A Treatise on Gun-shot Wounds: Written for and Dedicated to the Surgeons of the Confederate States Army* (New Orleans, 1861)

10. J.H. Packard: *A Manual of Minor Surgery* (Philadelphia, 1863)

11. Adjutant-General and the Surgeon-General: *List of Battles and Roster of Regimental Surgeons and Assistant Surgeons During the War of the Rebellion* (Washington, D.C., 1883)

A PRACTICAL TREATISE ON MILITARY SURGERY

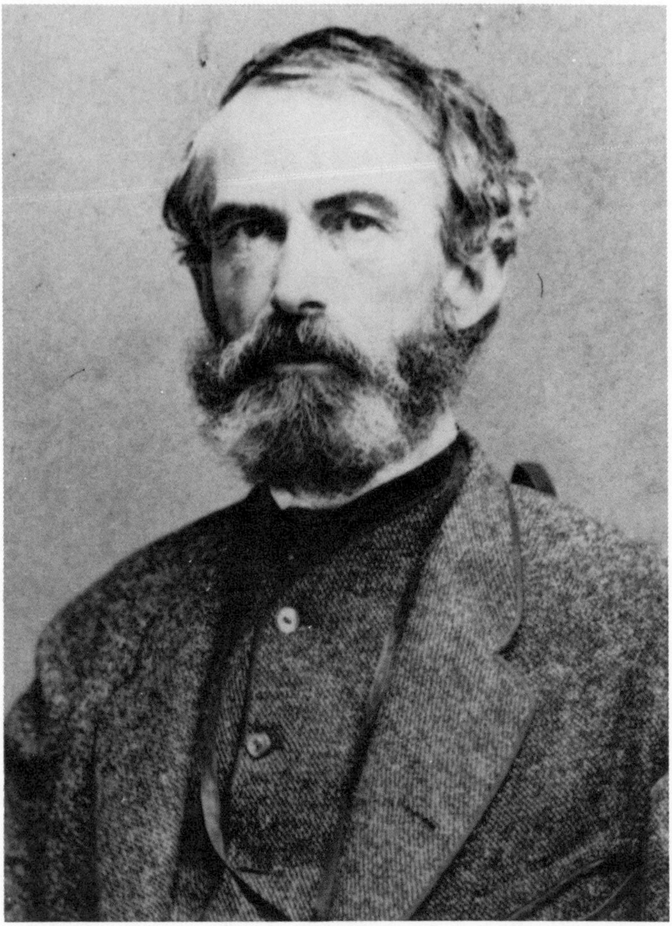

Frank Hastings Hamilton
1813–1886
National Library of Medicine

A PRACTICAL TREATISE ON MILITARY SURGERY

by

Frank Hastings Hamilton, M.D.

Reprinted with a Biographical Introduction

by Ira M. Rutkow, M.D., Dr.P.H.

Norman Publishing
San Francisco
1989

Published by Norman Publishing
Division of Jeremy Norman & Co., Inc.
442 Post Street
San Francisco, California 94102–1579

Library of Congress Cataloging-in-Publication Data

Hamilton, Frank Hastings, 1813–1886.
A practical treatise on military surgery.

(American Civil War surgery series ; no. 5)
Reprint. Originally published: New York :
Baillière, 1861.
1. Surgery, Military. I. Title. II. Series.
[DNLM: WO H217pa 1861a]
RD151.H25 1988 617'.99 88–60873
ISBN 0–930405–05–6 (alk. paper)

The American Civil War Surgery Series, No. 5

This book is printed on acid-free paper, and its binding materials have been chosen for strength and durability.

Manufactured in the United States of America.

Frank Hastings Hamilton

Frank Hastings Hamilton was born in Wilmington, Vermont, on September 10, 1813, the second son of Calvin and Lucinda Hamilton. His parents were farmers and also owned a local stagecoach line. For unknown reasons his family moved to Schenectady, New York, in 1816, and there Hamilton attended the Lancasterian School and the Schenectady Academy. He was an exceptional student and at age fourteen entered the sophomore class of Union College. Union was the first nondenominational college in the United States and was considered one of the foremost institutions of higher education in nineteenth-century America. Its liberal arts curriculum was quite comprehensive, and Hamilton there developed an interest in the classics that was later reflected in his work.

Hamilton graduated from Union in 1830 and registered as a private student of medicine with John Morgan, who was physician-surgeon to the state prison in Auburn, New York. During his three years of study with Morgan, Hamilton gained an education in the practice and fundamental principles of medicine. His greatest interest was in anatomy, which he was able to pursue through numerous dissections of recently deceased prisoners. As a consequence of this work he was able to paint life-size oils of nearly every part of the human body. During 1831 he attended a full course of lectures at the Western College of Physicians and Surgeons at Fairfield, New York. Although he received a license to practice medicine in 1833 from the Cayuga

County Medical Censors, Hamilton decided instead to obtain a formal medical degree from the University of Pennsylvania. He completed this work and graduated in 1835.

Hamilton returned to Auburn after graduation and began to give private instruction in anatomy and surgery. His work was well-received, and the 26-year-old Hamilton was unanimously appointed professor of surgery at the Western College in January 1839. Nineteen months later, in August 1840, he was given the chair of surgery in the Medical College at Geneva, New York. Hamilton remained at the institution for eight years, although he interrupted his work at Geneva for seven months in 1843–44 for travel and study in Europe. His European trip supplied materials for a diary, which soon appeared in the *Buffalo Medical Journal.*

After returning to Geneva, Hamilton decided in 1846 to accept a joint appointment as professor of surgery at Buffalo Medical College and surgeon to the Buffalo Charity Hospital. He held professorships at both Geneva and Buffalo for two years, resigning from Geneva in 1848 to attend more fully to his rapidly growing practice in Buffalo.

In Buffalo, Hamilton became friends with Austin Flint, Sr., (1812–86) and James Platt White (1811–81). Together they founded a medical department within the University of Buffalo and Hamilton was named professor of surgery and the first dean of the medical faculty. His career in Buffalo blossomed, and he soon became politically active in the profession with election to the presidency of the New York State Medical Society in 1855.

Hamilton remained in Buffalo until 1860, when he joined the newly organized faculty as professor of the principles and practice of surgery at the Long Island College Hospital in Brooklyn. In

May 1861 Hamilton was appointed to a special faculty position on military surgery. This was the earliest chair of military surgery in the country. Its establishment was closely related to the outbreak of the Civil War and the need for greater expertise in the management of traumatic wounds. With the commencement of hostilities, Hamilton entered the Army of the Potomac as surgeon to the Thirty-First Infantry of New York, also known as the Montezuma Battalion. While with the Thirty-First he was in charge of a field hospital during the First Battle of Bull Run. He remained with the regiment until September 1861. A year later he was promoted to corps surgeon and in the same year organized the army's Central Park General Hospital in New York. In 1863 Hamilton was appointed medical inspector of the United States Army with a rank of lieutenant-colonel. He continued in active service until September 1863, when he resigned his commission. While in the army he participated in a number of field campaigns and was captured twice: first by a party of Texas Rangers in Tennessee and later by a Confederate unit in Kentucky. He was well treated by the Confederates, who released him in both cases after a short period of internment.

In 1861 Hamilton had joined a group of physicians who helped found the Bellevue Hospital Medical College, where he was named professor of military surgery and fractures and dislocations. Hamilton took up the appointment on resigning his military commission and remained at the school in this capacity until 1868. After the retirement of James Rushmore Wood (1813–82) in that year, Hamilton assumed the key position of professor of the principles and practice of surgery. He held this post until his resignation in March 1875. However, he retained his position as one of the surgeons to Bellevue Hospital and continued to conduct weekly surgical clinics.

Hamilton's career was notable for an influential body of written work, including *A Monograph on Strabismus* (1845), *A Practical Treatise on Fractures and Dislocations* (1860), *A Practical Treatise on Military Surgery* (1861), *The Principles and Practice of Surgery* (1872), and *Fracture of the Patella* (1880). He also edited the two-volume *Surgical Memoirs of the War of the Rebellion: Collected and Published by the United States Sanitary Commission* (1870–71). Among Hamilton's most important journal articles were those on deformities after fractures and one of the first descriptions of skin grafting as a treatment for ulcers (elkoplasty or anaplasty). He also wrote about medical ethics in *An Essay on the Struggle for Life Against Civilization, Luxury, and Aestheticism* (1882) and *Conversations between Drs. Warren and Putnam on the Subject of Medical Ethics: With an Account of the Medical Empiricisms of Europe and America* (1884).

Hamilton's *A Practical Treatise on Military Surgery* was intended to supply information on areas in surgery, medicine, and hygiene, which, although related to military practice, were usually not considered in general surgical works. A second and much enlarged edition (648 pages with 127 engravings) was published in 1865.

Always active in organized medicine, Hamilton was president of the New York Pathological Society (1866), the New York Medico-Legal Society (1876), the American Academy of Medicine (1878), and the New York Society of Medical Jurisprudence (1885). From 1880 to 1884 he was vice-president of the New York Academy of Medicine. In 1869 the trustees of Union College conferred upon him the degree of Doctor of Laws.

Because of the respect accorded his surgical skills, Hamilton was a consulting surgeon to President James Garfield (1831–81) after Garfield was injured in an assassination attempt. Garfield suffered a lingering septic course secondary to an abdominal gunshot wound. Hamilton was a conspicuous figure during the ordeal, remaining almost constantly in attendance until Garfield died. Hamilton's candor in later joining in the publication of a report which criticized the poor quality of medical care that Garfield received and the repercussions of this report have become part of American surgical lore.

Hamilton is remembered eponymically for Hamilton's pseudophlegmon (a trophic affection of the subcutaneous connective tissue marked by a circumscribed swelling which may become indurated and red but never suppurates), and for Hamilton's test (a rod touching both the acromion process and the outer condyle of the humerus in axillary dislocation of the shoulder).

Hamilton was said to have had discriminating social and literary tastes. He also assembled a large medical library, which was detailed in a 36-page catalogue published shortly after his death. The collection was eventually purchased by John B. Hamilton (1847–98), no relation to Frank Hastings. Hamilton's unique assemblage of surgical specimens was bequeathed to the Army Medical Museum.

Hamilton was married twice. His first wife was Mary Virginia McMurran, whom he married in October 1834. They had one son, Theodore B. Hamilton. Mary Hamilton died in April 1838. In September 1840 he married Mary Gertrude Hart. He had three children by his second wife, who died in July 1885. Only two children survived him: his son Theodore and daughter Mary.

In December 1885, Hamilton had severe and repeated pulmonary hemorrhage due to tuberculosis. For the next year and a half his health continued to deteriorate, and he died in his New York City

home on 32nd Street on August 11, 1886. Interment was at the Sleepy Hollow Cemetery in Tarrytown, New York.

A

PRACTICAL TREATISE

ON

MILITARY SURGERY.

BY

FRANK HASTINGS HAMILTON, M.D.,

LATE SURGEON THIRTY-THIRD REGIMENT, FOURTH BRIGADE, FOURTH DIVISION, NEW YORK STATE ARTILLERY; PROFESSOR OF MILITARY SURGERY, AND OF DISEASES AND ACCIDENTS INCIDENT TO BONES, IN BELLEVUE MEDICAL COLLEGE; SURGEON TO BELLEVUE HOSPITAL; PROFESSOR OF SURGERY, AND SURGEON-IN-CHIEF TO THE LONG ISLAND COLLEGE HOSPITAL; AUTHOR OF "TREATISE ON FRACTURES AND DISLOCATIONS."

NEW YORK:

BAILLIÈRE BROTHERS, 440 BROADWAY.

LONDON:
H. BAILLIERE,
219 REGENT ST.

MELBOURNE:
F. BAILLIERE.

PARIS:
J. B. BAILLIERE ET FILS,
RUE HAUTEFEUILLE.

MADRID:
B. BAILLY-BAILLIERE,
CALLE DEL PRINCIPE.

1861.

R. CRAIGHEAD,
Printer, Stereotyper, and Electrotyper,
Caxton Building,
81, 83, *and* 85 *Centre Street.*

TO HIS COLLEAGUES

AUSTIN FLINT, JAMES D. TRASK, R. OGDEN DOREMUS, JOSEPH C. HUTCHISON, JOHN C. DALTON, DEWITT C. ENOS, EDWIN N. CHAPMAN,
Of the Long Island College Hospital:

AND

JAMES R. WOOD, LEWIS A. SAYRE, ALEXANDER B. MOTT, STEPHEN SMITH, ISAAC E. TAYLOR, GEORGE T. ELLIOT, FORDYCE BARKER, BENJAMIN W. McCREADY, JOHN W. S. GOULEY, AUSTIN FLINT, R. OGDEN DOREMUS, AUSTIN FLINT, JR.
Of the Bellevue Hospital Medical College.

AS A TESTIMONY OF ESTEEM,

THIS VOLUME IS RESPECTFULLY DEDICATED BY

The Author.

CONTENTS.

PREFACE.

The purpose of this volume is to supply information upon those points in Surgery, Medicine, and Hygiene, which, as having relation especially to military and naval practice, are usually not considered in general treatises. In so far, it is intended to be complete. Yet the author will not conceal his apprehensions that a more careful revision of the sheets than he has been able to give them, will disclose, even in this respect, serious omissions and perhaps other grave defects.

The author has to offer his grateful acknowledgments to Drs. Satterlee, Wood, Coolidge, Tripler, Mills, Pitcher, Wright, and others, of the U. S. Army; and to Drs. Parsons, Bache, Lockwood, Turner, Williams, and others, of the Navy, for many courtesies which have greatly facilitated his labors, and aided in the rapid completion of his work.

To Dr. Austin Flint, Professor of the Practice of Medicine in Bellevue and Long Island Hospital Colleges, and to Dr. Benjamin W. McCready, Professor of Materia Medica in Bellevue Medical College, the author is under especial obligations for the original chapters contributed by these two gentlemen respectively upon the subjects of Dysentery and Scurvy. The distinguished positions long occupied by Drs. Flint and McCready render it unnecessary to explain why they were selected to perform this part of the labor.

Gramercy Park, N.Y., May 28, 1861.

MILITARY SURGERY.

CHAPTER I.

INTRODUCTION.

Being a Discourse delivered by the Author at the Opening of a Course of Lectures on Military Surgery, at Bellevue Medical College, New York, April, 1861.

GENTLEMEN:—War is the normal condition of mankind; peace is the abnormal condition. This statement is not flattering to a people claiming Christianity and boasting of its civilization; it is nevertheless true, and the fact must be accepted. History is little else than a record of the contentions, conflicts, and conquests of nations. The sword and the cross, conventional emblems of battle-fields, stand as thick upon the round surface of the terrestrial sphere as stars upon the surface of the celestial. Each year, and almost every month in the year, commemorates some new achievement of arms, and places a new symbol upon the map; so that now, in the middle of the nineteenth century, as when Isaiah wrote, it is only in prophetic vision that we see the approach of that happy day when "swords shall be beaten into ploughshares and spears into pruning-hooks, and nations shall not learn war any more."

We must not be surprised, therefore, that a great part of mankind have occupied themselves, and still continue to occupy themselves, in the improvement and perfection of the art of war; nor that it has come at last to take rank almost among the exact sciences. It has been the study especially of kings, princes, governors, statesmen, philosophers, and military chieftains, who have created for it a factitious, but universally conceded, nobility, by virtue of which it takes precedence of all other sciences, while it condescends, in order to the attainment of its selfish ends, to impress them into its service.

But surgery, like many other departments of knowledge which have been compelled to submit to this tyranny, and to contribute reluctantly to the perfection of a barbarous art, has, in its application to the purposes of war, we are happy to say, other and more legitimate ends. It is equally the mission of the Military Surgeon to prevent, as far as possible, all useless expenditure of life. In civilized warfare life is spared whenever a firelock is grounded, or an arm is disabled; and, so well is this understood, the wounded soldier does not hesitate to throw himself upon the mercy of his captors for surgical aid, since he is equally certain of receiving succor from the surgical corps of a foe as of a friend. Consider how much this serves to soften the savage aspect of war; that if battles must be fought, the results should be obtained with as little sacrifice of life, with as little mutilation and suffering as possible. The world, gentlemen, is indebted to our profession for this.

At the same time, also, many excellent surgeons bring away from these great schools of practice valuable lessons of experience, which, being carefully written down, are of service to those who live after them. Waterloo, Sevastopol, and Solferino, witnessed each a terrible slaughter of human beings; but let us hope that in the faithful "annals of their sufferings," recorded by Larrey, Guthrie, Hennen, Armand, and others, the world will find some compensation, if not actual occasion for gratitude, since they have added so many new fasciculi to our stores of knowledge; and since it is not impossible the lives which will be thereby saved will outnumber the lives which were lost in those battles." "It is one of the happy privileges of the military surgeon," says Armand, "to draw from the state of war precepts which console humanity, by turning to his profit the observations and the treatment of the maladies which follow in its train."

Military and naval surgery is not a new and distinct science, but only the science of medicine in its largest sense, with a special application. The principles of civil and military surgery are the same, or nearly the same; but the application of those principles is varied or modified, according to the varying exigencies of the case. Anatomy, physiology, chemistry, botany, and pharmacy, lie at the foundation of each; and what of these has been learned in the schools is equally applicable to both. So also the sciences of military practice, military surgery, and military hygiene, are nearly identical in their fundamental laws with the civil sciences so named; but they differ occasionally in their subordinate rules; more often in their modes of procedure, and in the use of means by which they seek to accomplish the same ends. But perhaps the widest difference will be found to consist in the relative frequency of certain accidents and diseases; insomuch that what is of daily occurrence, and a common experience in the one, is rarely seen in the other, and the reverse.

A few examples will illustrate these important differences. It is well known that certain conditions of the limb generally demand amputation in military practice; as, for example, a gunshot wound traversing a large joint; while the same conditions do not necessarily exact the same sacrifice in civil practice. This change or modification of the rule evidently has reference to the altered condition of treatment to which the soldier and civilian will probably be subjected.

In civil practice, the time occupied in any operation, especially since the introduction of anæsthetics, is generally regarded as a matter of secondary importance. And that mode which possesses even trifling points of superiority with reference to the final result, even though more tedious in its execution, justly claims the preference. Here we may properly apply the maxim, "sat cito, si sat bene." But in military practice, at least in most operations made upon the field, and where, as is usually the case, the number of surgeons is small in proportion to the number of wounded, time is of the first importance, and minor preferences must yield to major necessities. It will not do to let one man die of hæmorrhage from the femoral artery because you wish to apply a ligature very methodically to the ulnar artery of another; nor to amputate a limb by circular incisions, when by oval incisions it can be done in half the time. Armand, whose noble sentiments one is frequently compelled to admire, speaking of his experience as surgeon to the ambulance of the Imperial Guard during the Crimean war, observes, "In ordinary times of the siege, the local barracks, or the tents, sufficed. In the grand engagements, the encumbrance of the wounded was such that it became necessary to gather them into groups here and there; and God knows, then, how painful was the mission of the surgeons, who were compelled to multiply themselves to succor the hundreds, the thousands of the wounded constantly imploring their aid!" There was but one precept then, "*Cite!* citissime!"

Broken limbs, when dressed in the midst of an engagement, cannot exact the same amount of care and attention in their adjustment as in a well supplied hospital, or as in ordinary private practice. The appliances must be simple, few, and, in many cases, measurably inadequate. They must be adapted especially to the conditions requisite for transportation. Complicated double-inclined planes, pulleys, and swings, however useful they might be for limbs at rest, are wholly inapplicable to those cases in which the patient has to be transported long distances in wagons and over rough roads. The most enthusiastic advocate of Pott's treatment of broken limbs, without side splints or extension, would never be so absurd as to claim for it a preference under these circumstances.

General treatises upon surgery and surgical teachers, assume that both the patient and his medical attendant are placed always under the most favorable circumstances: that ample time is allowed for a careful diagnosis; and, in view of an operation, that the patient is brought up to the best possible condition of preparation: that he is at least comfortably lodged, suitably nourished, and that his surgeon has at his command all the instruments and appliances which can render the execution of the operation more easy, and its success more certain. No man who has had much experience in teaching, and in examining medical students, can have failed to notice the danger of suggesting inferior alternatives for exceptional cases, which, through inattention or carelessness, are often substituted in the minds of the pupil for the general law; and it is with much propriety, therefore, that these omissions are generally made.

It is the special province of military and naval surgery to supply these deficiencies; instructing the pupil how, by a multitude of extemporaneous expedients, he may succor the wounded and relieve the sick when the usual resources fail or are not at hand; how he may make the products of every country contribute to his necessities, and a single cruse of oil minister miraculously to a thousand.

As we have intimated, however, the widest difference between civil and military surgery is to be found in the relative frequency of certain accidents and diseases. Club-feet, rickets, hip-disease, and strabismus, are of every-day occurrence in domestic and city hospital practice, while they are almost unknown to army practice. On the other hand, scurvy, gunshot, sword, and bayonet wounds are rarely met with in the first, while they are common in the second.

Such as remain sceptical upon this point have only to enter successively, the wards of a military and of a civil hospital; to compare with each other a civil and a military dispensary; or examine the private records of a civil and of a military surgeon, to convince themselves that the two schools do not furnish, relatively, the same instruction.

In order to be prepared, also, for all the duties imposed upon an army surgeon, one must understand what are the peculiar physical qualifications necessary to become an efficient soldier—what conditions imply health, endurance, agility, and we may add, courage. It is the first part of a surgeon's duty to select and arrange the tools by which the work is to be done, and the remainder of his duty is to keep these tools in order.

Will any one say that our services are unimportant, and our position a subordinate one in the business of war? The fact is, that neither tactics nor strategy will serve an army of invalids. These men perish or are demoralized when no enemy is opposed to them; and more than one campaign, which opened auspiciously, has been brought to a disastrous close in consequence of the injudicious selection of recruits, and of the lack of suitable provisions on the part of the government or of the officers for the preservation of their health. The mortifying termination of several campaigns, especially at the North, during the war of 1812 in this country, sufficiently demonstrates the truth of these assertions.

Feigned diseases, also, need to be studied. They bear the same relations, in military surgery, to actual diseases, as sophisticated drugs bear to the genuine; and to occupy a position of trust in the medical staff of the army, without some knowledge of the ingenious dissimulations practised by soldiers to relieve themselves from duty, or to obtain a discharge and a pension, would be as unjust to the public whom you serve as to undertake the duties of a pharmaceutist or of a drug-inspector, without any competent knowledge of the art of sophistication.

The diet, dress, and general hygiene of the troops; the transport of the sick and wounded; the construction and location of tents, barracks, and hospitals, with a view to their healthfulness; the arrangement of bivouacs; are among the subjects which properly belong to this branch of surgery.

Finally, as not the least valuable of those accomplishments which ought to adorn an army medical officer, we must not omit to enumerate a thorough knowledge of geography, climatology, meteorology, geology, and botany, with many other kindred subjects belonging to the natural sciences.

Remember, gentlemen, that when you enter the army or the navy of the United States, you will be brought into immediate association with a body of highly educated and polished gentlemen. It is one distinction of the American military system which the English have not yet reached, that every commissioned officer of the line has attained his position, not by purchase, by nepotism, or by any other species of favoritism, but only through a regular curriculum, passed in either the army or navy schools, established under authority of the government, at West Point and Annapolis.

If the citizens of the United States of America may justly feel proud of the high character which the officers of the line, both in the army and navy, have acquired at home and abroad; we have no less reason to feel proud of the honorable distinction which our army and naval medical boards have acquired by the rigor of their examinations; and through them, of the recognised elevated standing of its medical officers. No one has been admitted to the rank of Assistant Surgeon, or been promoted to the rank of Surgeon in the American regular service, for many years, who did not possess the most eminent qualifications, both medical and literary, for those positions; nor are they likely hereafter to abate the stringency of their demands, as you will probably learn if you ever go before them for examination.

While improvements are being constantly made in the construction of firearms and of other weapons of warfare, and the art of war is advancing step by step towards the complete attainment of its purpose, it is delightful to observe how steadily, yet silently, the genius of medicine follows upon its heavy tread. The introduction of gunpowder as an instrument of war, was soon followed by the discovery and application of the ligature to wounded arteries after amputations. So that if thereafter the soldiers were not permitted to escape the terrible wounds inflicted by bullets and "fiery balls," they were saved from the more appalling infliction of having their mutilated stumps plunged into boiling pitch, to arrest the bleeding. And in our own day, the conical bullet and the rifled cannon have been overtaken by the discovery of the anæsthetic properties of chloroform and of ether.

The establishment of flying or field ambulances has also contributed greatly to the amelioration of the condition of the soldier, and, it may be said, to the efficiency of the service.

They are usually composed of the medical staff and picked men, who hang upon the rear, and press themselves into the very shadow of the advancing columns; and while the surgeons, with their assistants, stationed here and there in places of partial security, are prepared to render prompt surgical aid, the men who are especially charged with that duty, bring the wounded in panniers and upon litters to the several regimental depots.

The practice of employing field ambulances is now almost universal, but the plan of organization is much varied by different nations.

Richter, Physician General to the 8th corps of the Prussian army, who has devoted much attention to this subject, and to whose suggestions the Prussian army is indebted for its present excellent system of field ambulances, informs us that Austria, ever since the Italian and Hungarian campaigns, in 1848 and 1849, has employed with great success "*des troupes de santé*," and that this institution has been imitated in Bavaria, Saxony, and Hanover.

The Prussian system, established by royal ordinance in 1854, may serve as a model, or as an example most deserving of imitation. The "*Compagnies des porte-malades*," as they are sometimes called, are composed of one captain, three lieutenants, three assistant surgeons, with the rank of lieutenants; two hundred and three men, of which seventeen are non-commissioned officers, including a sergeant-major and a quartermaster; sixteen exempts (premiers soldats) and six *clairons.*

Each company is divided into three squads, that is to say, one squad for each hospital ambulance of the three grand divisions of the army. Each squad is composed of ten officers and one assistant surgeon, each of which is furnished with two horses; five non-commissioned officers, sixty soldiers and exempts, and two *clairons.*

Each squad has fifteen litters, equal to forty-five for the whole company.

In the American service the system of flying ambulances is less complete and perfect in its details. The only assistance which a regimental surgeon and his adjuncts can claim upon the field of battle, is that of the band, and of a hospital orderly, who, by an order of the army board, made in November, 1859, is required to accompany the medical officer whether upon the march or in the field; the orderly carrying upon his back a knapsack, in which are placed such instruments, dressings, and medicines as may be needed in an emergency.

As to the value and importance of a well regulated system of field ambulances, it might be sufficient to say, that all of the army surgeons are agreed upon this subject, and its claims have been repeatedly urged by Percy, Hennen, Guthrie, Larrey, Jackson, Armand, Richter, Mann, and others, and that by most of the enlightened governments of Europe they have been adopted and carried out to an admirable degree of perfection.

But since the government of the United States has been slow to accept of all the improvements in this department, introduced and now fairly tested abroad, it will be proper to enumerate some of their advantages.

It will not be denied that humanity, and a just policy of economy, dictate that the wounded should receive succor as soon as possible, and that for this purpose the surgeons, with their assistants, ought to be stationed as near to the field of action as is consistent with their own safety, and the safety of those who are under their charge; nor will it be doubted that soldiers and officers will be less reluctant to expose themselves to the hazards of a battle when they feel assured that competent surgical aid is at hand. Whatever may be a man's apparent disregard of life, experience shows that most men, even when in heat, would of the two, rather kill their antagonist than die themselves. To be wounded may be honorable, but to die perchance is unnecessary. And better soldiers than Falstaff—nor is it any reflection upon their courage to say so—have probably uttered his soliloquy upon the eve of battle: "Can honor set to a broken leg? No. Or an arm? No. Or take away the grief of a wound? No. Honor hath no skill in surgery, then? No."

There is a single incident in the life of Ambrose Paré, which, having been often mentioned by historical writers, is probably familiar to you all, but which, as furnishing a pertinent illustration of the confidence inspired in a whole army by the immediate presence of a skilful surgeon, merits a repetition at this time.

The ancient city of Metz was at one time besieged by an army of one hundred thousand men, commanded by Charles the Fifth in person. Within the walls were gathered a multitude of men, including nearly all the princes and nobility of France. Decimated by famine, disease, and by wounds received in the protracted defence, the garrison were reduced almost to extremities. At this critical juncture the king sent to them his own surgeon, the great

Paré, who had been successively surgeon to four kings of France, and who had during this period followed the French armies in all their campaigns. He was introduced into the city at night, by an Italian captain, and on the following morning being requested by the governor to show himself upon the breach, he was received by the soldiers with shouts of triumph. "We shall not die," they exclaimed, "even though wounded—Paré is among us!" From this time the defence was conducted with renewed vigor; and to the presence of this single man it has been universally conceded that the city was indebted for its salvation, although the siege was not raised until "the gallant army which lay around it had perished beneath its walls."

The value of medical services to an army, in a strategic, economical, and humane point of view, is indisputable.

The only real question then is as to the best mode of getting the soldiers wounded in battle to the hospital depots.

A considerable proportion find no difficulty in reaching the depots without assistance; and it is wonderful sometimes through how small a wound a large amount of courage will ooze out. The slightest prick of a bayonet or the loss of a finger will cripple some men and send them halting to the rear. These soldiers will take care of themselves.

But when a man falls who is seriously wounded, and not killed outright, it is a common practice in both the American and British service for the officer in command to order a couple of soldiers to carry him off. This withdraws three men from the line instead of one. But unfortunately it is well known that soldiers do not always wait for this authority. The commanding officer is not always where he can observe the conduct of all of his men; and impelled by the instinct of humanity, they, in many instances, cheerfully anticipate the supposed wishes of their officers, and seizing their fallen comrade they bear him hastily from the field. The effect of this is most demoralizing; for while it actually and materially diminishes the force of the column, it diverts the attention of the soldiers and of the officers from their first purpose, especially by substituting the more delicate and enervating sentiments of humanity for those coarser but more stimulating passions, revenge and ambition, by which the courage of troops is chiefly sustained.

Ballingall says: "We find the Duke of Wellington, in his general order, cautioning the commanding officers of regiments, and the officers and non-commissioned officers of companies, to take care that no man falls out of the ranks under pretence of assisting the wounded, when he is not ordered to do so by his officer;" and Mr. Alcock states that he has seen "in less than an hour, a whole battalion tail off after some fifty wounded."

There are many circumstances under which the escape of the wounded soldier from the mêlée of the conflict is impossible; and in which the incessant pressure of troops from the rear presents no alternative but to be trodden under foot by men and horses, or to be crushed by the wheels of the cannon. If, however, the storm of battle has in some measure passed over, and the wounded man is on that side of the clouds from which the rainbow can be seen —and it is to such alone that assistance can ever be offered —then he may be easily rescued by the soldiers of the ambulance, and borne upon a litter to a place of safety. The army will, in this way, be separated into two distinct yet very disproportionate bodies; the one being occupied solely in killing, maiming, and mutilating, and the other in ministering to the sufferings of the wounded: thus no infection will be communicated from one to the other, and the morale of both will be preserved.

It is with some reluctance that we shall call your attention to other subjects, having no very intimate relation to the general theme of our discourse, yet possessing a peculiar interest in their relations to the public service, the profession of medicine generally, and the medical gentlemen of the army. We allude to the subjects of rank and of authority.

Ever since the establishment of a medical department in connexion with armies, or until within a very recent period, it has been customary to consider and hold the medical officers, of whatever grade, as subordinate to the other branches of the service—conferring upon them neither rank nor authority in any case. The practice has been thought to be unjust to an honorable profession, and of doubtful utility to the public interest; and from time to time the subject has been pressed upon the consideration of the various governments by distinguished army surgeons, both in this country and upon the continent of Europe, whose representations have had the effect, in many cases, of bringing about certain manifest improvements, although they have failed anywhere to accomplish all that is desired.

In relation to *rank*, probably the most decided step in advance has been made in our own country by the Act of Congress approved Feb. 11, 1847, which declares that, "the rank of the officers of the Medical Department of the Army, shall be arranged upon the same basis which at present determines the amount of their pay and emoluments: Provided, that medical officers shall not, in virtue of such rank, be entitled to command in the line or other staff departments of the army."

This was a well considered and enlightened act of legislation, intended to remove the medical officers from that position of subordination where they had so long been subject to petty annoyances, and even to the insults of inferior officers of the line, and to secure for them those courtesies, and that respect, which they had a right to claim. It conferred no authority to command, nor any privileges which one gentleman should ever hesitate to concede to another; but it is well known that, from the time of the passage of this act until the present moment, a few officers of the army and navy have persistently refused to recognise its obligations, and that they habitually and openly violate both its spirit and its letter.

We wish especially to exonerate from this charge the great body of the army and navy officers, by whom the medical officers have been uniformly treated with the greatest courtesy. The exceptions, however, have been found to be sufficiently numerous, in which the officers of the line have refused to comply with the law, to call forth repeated remonstrances from the surgeons, and to render it proper in the opinion of Surgeon-General Lawson to issue a circular, recommending to medical officers a conciliatory but decided stand, reminding them that "encroachment promptly met will be more promptly checked; while any evidence of irresolution, or want of confidence in the correctness of their position, might lead to further aggression."

We understand those who refuse a compliance with the law to say, in justification, that surgeons are non-combatants, and that to combatants alone, upon whom, they affirm, rest the hazards and responsibilities of war, rightly belong its honors.

This distinction has been made before, and it has been

the constant pretext for opposition to the conferring of rank upon medical officers; yet we deny that it has any foundation in fact, and it is plainly calculated, if it is not intended, to depreciate our position and to underrate our service. Says Dr. Tripler: "The old distinction between combatants and non-combatants, as applied to the medical officer, has been roughly handled, and in not a few instances scouted as absurd, by officers of the highest rank in the British army. In our own army they are the only officers of the administrative branches of the general staff whose duties require them to be present on the field of battle. In the brilliant campaign of Gen. Scott in Mexico, the medical staff was the only one that had an officer killed or wounded. No officer of the Quartermaster or Subsistence Department was either killed or wounded. To any one who understands the meaning of terms, and the duties of these departments, to call one of them combatants in contradistinction to the other, as a pretext for conferring military rank upon that one and denying it to the other, is simply absurd. We may say as Cicero did of the Roman augurs: 'We cannot see how two men, maintaining that opinion, can look each other in the face without laughing.'" Dr. Tripler properly adds: "Inveterate habit in the abuse of terms has drifted us thus far unresistingly with the notion that the Commissary of Subsistence, who purchases provisions in Cincinnati for the subsistence of the soldiers, is a combatant, while a medical officer is officially a non-combatant."

If exposure to hardship and danger is to be the ground upon which rank is to be conceded to officers of the army or of the navy, we think the claim of the medical officers may be easily determined. The medical officers are exposed to the same hardships on the march or in cantonment as the officers of the line; and while the latter have to incur the hazards of battle only occasionally, perhaps but once in a campaign, the former may be said to be doing battle daily, being constantly subjected to the dangers of pestilence by their exposure to the contagions and infections of crowded and unwholesome hospitals. We have not the statistics before us upon which to base a positive statement, but we entertain little doubt that, were the facts known, it would be found that in proportion to the number employed in any campaign, the number of deaths, or of invalided in the medical staff, by the ordinary casualties and exposures of the service, is greater than in any other department.

But as compared with the quartermaster or subsistence officers, the hazards of the medical officers are undeniably greater. The services of the first are never required upon the field; while the surgeons are expected to accompany their respective regiments until the action commences—and then only to retire to some position of comparative, but not absolute safety. The instances upon record in which medical officers have been wounded and killed upon the field of battle, when in discharge of their appropriate duties, are numerous. In savage warfare very little respect is usually paid to any theoretical distinctions between combatants and non-combatants; and in civilized warfare the distinction is by no means constantly observed by an excited and disorderly soldiery.

Surgeon Dunigan, writing from the Crimea during the siege of Sevastopol, states, "already one medical officer has been killed and two or three wounded. The first, Mr. O'Leary, Assistant Surgeon of the 68th Regiment of Light Infantry, was actually cut in two by a cannon-ball while in the act of assisting a wounded seaman. It is only to be wondered at that more casualties have not occurred among the medical officers, for during the heat of the fire they are constantly called from place to place, running along the batteries, through the line of fire, in quest of the wounded. During the second bombardment this peripatetic system was very trying and fatiguing, for the soil was heavy and tenacious from the torrents of rain that then deluged the trenches; and instances occurred where officers' boots drew off while running along to assist the wounded * * * "On the whole," he remarks, "this trench duty is very trying and hazardous; and in performing it, the medical men run the same dangers, if not more, certainly not less, than the executive officers, who are generally stationary in a battery, while the medical officer, as ubiquitous as possible, is rushing in all directions to succor the wounded."*

Dr. Jarvis, surgeon in the U. S. Army, in a letter dated Oct., 1846, describing the attack upon Monterey, says— "The nearest and only shelter that presented itself to me for the wounded, falling every moment under a most destructive fire, was a quarry-pit, four or five feet in depth, and the same in breadth. Several of these were contiguous, and to them I directed the wounded to be carried. By stooping we were protected from the shots, which, however, became every moment thicker, owing to the fact that our troops had by this time advanced within range of the enemy's fire, and the moment they perceived a party of men bringing the wounded to us, they directed all their guns upon it. I had already performed one amputation, and was preparing for a second, when two or three fugitives rushed into the pit, falling over the wounded that lay there crowded together, saying that a large body of lancers were approaching. So little credit did I attach to their

* New York Journal of Medicine, vol. 15, 2d series, p. 424, from Medical Times and Gazette.

report, which I ascribed rather to their fears than to the actual presence of this dreaded description of troops, that I never raised my eyes to observe them, which circumstance doubtless saved us all. Had I been discovered, all would have been massacred, as in their headlong fury they would neither have delayed to ascertain our character or profession, nor have paid much respect to our patients. Several soldiers who had sought an adjoining pit, with an officer, were slain."

Several times, subsequently, during the engagement, Dr. Jarvis was compelled to change his quarters, owing to the constant and heavy fire which was kept up on the parties approaching with the wounded, whenever they were discovered by the enemy. And although it is true that the ambulance flag is generally respected, yet this, with many other similar examples to which we are prepared to refer, sufficiently shows that the exceptions are not rare.

The life of Larrey was frequently exposed to the most imminent hazards upon the field of battle. At Waterloo, he was taken prisoner, and was upon the point of being shot, after having being robbed of his watch and purse, when he was recognised by a Prussian surgeon, and his life saved.

We wish, moreover, to remind the officers of the executive department of the army, that while there are many points of antagonism between their duties and those of the medical department, there are also some points of parallelism, and such as ought to suggest a sympathy and fraternity of feeling. If bravery is a quality of excellence in those who call themselves the "fighting men," when have medical men, either in or out of the army, shown themselves cowards? Not at Norfolk; not at Sandusky; not at Bellevue; nor anywhere else, so far as we know. Napoleon always called his medical officers "my brave surgeons;' and we believe that no class is less amenable to the charge of cowardice than medical men generally. They are trained in a Spartan school, under, if we may so term it, a law of ethics which allows no man to turn his back upon danger. Whatever may be the peril, they are expected to go wherever their services are needed. They make no great ado about it; nor are their names often mentioned in the official reports; and still less often are they breveted for soldier-like conduct; yet they go, wherever they are called, quietly about their business, alone or in small detachments, in rain and in snow, by night and by day, on the march and on the bivouac, through watchfulness, and fasting, and fatigue, into the midst of malaria, contagion, and battle.

We challenge any man to-day to point us to an educated physician who has fled at the approach of pestilence, or who has hesitated to enter the trenches, or to face the batteries, if required to do so, in the performance of his legitimate duties. Even when the strict letter of his instructions forbade his exposure, the medical officer has seldom been backward to accept any duty which the exigency seemed to impose upon him.

In this way fell, at the terrible slaughter of El Molino del Rey, on the 8th of Sept., 1847, the author's beloved pupil, George Wm. Roberts, Assistant-Surgeon in the 5th Regt. U. S. Infantry. Having received from the Staff Surgeon no authority to retire (an omission which, in the confusion of the onset, may be readily explained), he continued at the head of his regiment until nearly all the officers had fallen, when he begged permission from Capt. Hamilton, who was at that moment disabled by a wound in the shoulder, to be allowed to lead the broken column. Permission was granted, there being no officer of the line left to succeed in the command; and in a moment after Roberts received a wound through his head which proved fatal; but his death did not occur until several days after the battle, and when he had received at the hands of his comrades all the attention and care which their affection for him could suggest.

It is with pleasure that we refer those who deny the medical officers such courtesies as a law of Congress has instructed the officers of the line to observe, to the views of one who is in no way connected with the medical profession, and whose opinions, from the position of isolation and independence which he occupies, will be entitled to respect. Lord Dalhousie, in a memoir upon the Medical Service, appended to the Report of the Parliamentary Committee, remarks as follows:

"There are several particulars in which the Medical Service, as a body, lies under great disadvantages, and which they regard, justly in my opinion, as grievances that ought to be removed. I refer to the inequality which now prevails between the position of a medical officer and that of his brother officers, in respect of pension, honor, and rank. I respectfully submit that such inequalities are founded on no sound grounds of justice, expediency, or policy; no valid reason ever has been, or can be, alleged for maintaining them. Their effect is to depress the spirit of the medical officers, to depreciate a profession and class of service which ought to be held in the utmost respect, and supported equally from motives of prudence and gratitude.

"But the most galling, the most unmeaning, and purposeless regulations by which a sense of inferiority is imposed upon medical officers, is by the refusal to them of *substantive rank.* The surgeon and assistant-surgeon rank invariably with captain and lieutenant, but the rank is only *nominal;* whenever medical officers and others are brought together on public duty, the former have no rank at all, and the oldest surgeon on the list must, in such case, range himself below the youngest ensign last posted to a corps.

"It is impossible to conceive how such a system as this can have been maintained so long on the strength of no better argument than that it has been, and therefore ought to be! It is impossible to imagine what serious justification can be offered for a system which, in respect to external position, postpones service to inexperience, cunning to ignorance, age to youth; a system which gives a subaltern who is hardly free from his drill, precedence over his elder, who perhaps has served through every campaign for thirty years; a system which treats a member of a learned profession, a man of ability, skill, and experience, as inferior in position to a cornet of cavalry, just entering on his study of the pass and audit regulations; a system, in fine, which thrusts down grey-headed veterans below beardless boys."

The only remaining point to which we wish to call your attention is the amount of *authority* vested in the medical officers of the army, with a view to a consideration of the question whether it is sufficient for the purposes intended: and we may say at once, that it is the almost unanimous opinion of the army surgeons that it is not sufficient unless the medical officers have complete control of the medical department; in the same manner and to the same extent, that the officers of the corps of engineers control their department. In this opinion, the writer fully concurs.

The objections to conferring authority upon medical officers are the same which have been urged against medical rank; and in addition to these it has been claimed, that to divide or distribute authority, is to destroy the unity and power of the army, and that it is essentially destructive of all military discipline. The first of these objections has already been sufficiently considered, and the second is very well disposed of by Dr. Tripler in a few words: "The dogma of the necessary alternate of commanding or being commanded, that has been the fruitful source of so many mischiefs, and is at the root of the difficulty of securing the efficient co-operation of the different professions that are now combined in the organization of the army, has had its practical refutation demonstrated in our service by the experience of almost half a century. The law forbids the exercise of command, out of their corps, to the officers of the engineers. Still they are not subject to the orders of their juniors in the line. They cannot command, nor are they commanded except by a superior; and what has been the result of this assumed military heresy? Let the world produce their superiors as an efficient and scientific corps! Their independence of all outside interference, and their being exclusively intrusted with the means of performing their own duties, have made them what they are, and the country has reaped the advantages of its wise legislation in regard to them. This is the only corps in the army that has any analogy with the medical, as regards scientific acquirement, specialty of function, peculiarity of administration, and claims to independence of action, because it is not at all understood or comprehended by any other department."*

We conclude then, that to the medical officers ought to be intrusted the complete control of the medical department, because upon the preservation of the health of the troops

* Amer. Med. Gazette. Introduc. Lec. on Mil. Surg. By Charles S. Tripler, M.D., Surgeon U. S. A. (1848.)

depends in a great measure the success of every expedition; because no others than medical men are, by their education and habits, qualified to perform this duty; because no one else is competent to decide upon the proper location of a hospital, its construction, ventilation, or general arrangement; no one else can determine what is necessary for the sick, in the way of diet, clothing, medicines, etc.; no one else knows when rooms are overcrowded, and are in danger of becoming pestilential, or when patients can be removed with safety. In short, because officers of the executive department, from the entirely distinct nature of their pursuits, whatever they may believe to the contrary, do actually know as little of hygiene, medicine, and surgery, as they do of engineering. Because, moreover, medical men are supposed to be qualified, they are appointed for the express purpose, and because, without authority, they are unable to carry out their own views, and it is impossible, therefore, that the public service can receive the full benefit of their ability.

Fortunately, recent events in the Crimea and in Turkey have furnished an opportunity to test, in some degree, the relative value of the two systems as applied directly to the medical department.

The French army sanitary system is exceedingly complicated, and its details are made out in the most elaborate manner; nothing is left to conjecture; every duty is defined so explicitly that there can be no chance of error. As to authority to deviate from these rules, they have none. Each hospital is placed under the charge of an officer of the line, called the Military Intendant, whose only qualification for this position is that he possesses military rank, by virtue of which he is entitled to command. The medical officer merely prescribes and makes surgical operations, dresses wounds, and *suggests*. He cannot command the most subordinate attaché of the wards. He cannot, in theory, order a nurse to dispense a medicine, or a sick soldier to leave his bed, except through the Military Intendant.

In the British service, the system is much less elaborate, and there is much less precision in the rules which govern its details. So that, to the casual observer, it seems imperfect, and contrasts unfavorably with the French system; but the British surgeons are permitted to exercise a certain amount of authority over their own department, such as is not allowed to the French surgeons.

In the allied expedition against Russia, of 1856, the British medical officer had authority to command over the hospital orderlies, the nurses, and the apothecaries. He was permitted to regulate the general hospital police, to give orders, and to enforce their execution in relation to the hygiene, medication, and subsistence of the sick.

The result, fairly traceable to these apparently insignificant, but as every medical man knows them to be, important practical differences, was that the English army closed its campaign with a loss, by death or invaliding, of less than one-third of the troops, while the French had lost more than one-half of their whole number.

It must be understood also that by far the largest proportion of those who died or were invalided in these campaigns were thus lost to the service by epidemics, such as the cholera, dysentery, &c., which were in a great measure capable of prevention. The proportion lost by wounds received in battle was very small, probably not more than one in ten or fifteen.

Whether, as more than one writer has intimated, the French were compelled to make a hasty peace, because their forces were broken and disheartened by the progress of disease amongst them, we are not prepared to say; but however this may be, it is certainly capable of mathematical demonstration that without large additional conscriptions, and we may add, some change in the condition of the sanitary police of the army, the emperor would have been compelled soon to close the war on the part of France by a disgraceful retreat.

M. Baudens does not hesitate to declare the imperfection of the French regulations as contrasted with those of their English ally, and to intimate the real source of their own misfortunes. "The English hospitals," he remarks, "were remarkable for cleanliness. We have seen that this quality did not exist in ours. The difference is partly due to the higher and more independent military position which the English surgeon holds, and which entitles and enables him to exercise greater authority in hygienic measures. His ordinary sick-diet table is more ample and varied than the French, and the surgeon can order what extras he thinks proper for the sick. Indeed, the English camp was abundantly supplied with stores and comforts of all kinds; to which circumstance is to be ascribed its preservation from scurvy and typhus in 1856."

To the crowding of sick tents and huts into a confined area, in opposition to the protests of the army surgeons, both in the Crimea and at Constantinople, this writer ascribes the persistence of the cholera, and the prevalence and ravages of typhus and hospital gangrene. The army intendants and the medical officers entertained wholly different opinions as to what constituted overcrowding. The intendence functionaries "adhered to the strict letter of the military rule: so long as the patient had the regulation allowance of cubic feet, overcrowding was an impossibility; while physicians saw it to exist from the moment when disease was aggravated, and its fatality augmented by reason of too many sick being congregated within a given space."

What can be more conclusive? Admitting that some minor embarrassments might arise from an occasional collision of authority between co-ordinate branches; still is it not too plain to allow of a doubt, that to subordinate a department, with which are intrusted such vast interests, to a department wholly unacquainted with its duties, is to put the whole army in extreme peril, and to place the results of the expedition almost upon the hazards of a die?

The position which we assume, however, is that, so far as experience goes, there is no evidence that by rendering certain departments of the army co-ordinate the danger of collision is increased. On the contrary, we believe that by this method alone can collision be effectually prevented. They will have less contact, either personal, ceremonial, or official; consequently, we believe, there will be less jarring, less jealousy, less crimination, and more faithful service.

We trust, for the sake of humanity, that the War Department at Washington will listen to the respectful suggestions which are constantly being made by experienced army surgeons upon this subject; and that these suggestions will receive from them early and earnest consideration.

CHAPTER II.

EXAMINATION OF RECRUITS.

THE examination of recruits constitutes an important part of the duties of a military surgeon. Upon him depends the selection of the men who are to constitute the rank and file of the army. It is as necessary that the choice should be made judiciously as that the army should be supplied with proper weapons and suitable food. Writers upon military surgery have therefore given to this subject a good deal of attention, and nearly all governments have adopted regulations for the guidance of recruiting officers and boards of inspectors, differing somewhat according to the peculiar service in which the men are to be employed, the kind of weapons used, the length of time during which they are to serve, the genius of the people, and the exigencies under which the enlistments are made.

We shall endeavor to give, in this chapter, a general idea of what is required of those who enter the "regular army" of the United States of America by voluntary enlistment or by draft; being guided chiefly by the Manual prepared by Charles S. Tripler, Surgeon in the U. S. A., and which was published by authority of the Department of War, and its standards adopted in 1858.

It is proper to say that Dr. Tripler has taken as the basis of his Manual the "Aide-Memoire de l'Officier de Santé" for the French army, upon which, he acknowledges, that he has drawn freely; making only such changes as were necessary in order to adapt it to the American service, and such as his own experience and the observations of others seemed to demand.

It has been our plan also, while adhering to the strict letter of this excellent "guide," to condense the whole into a more compact form, and to add such suggestions as our own reading and observation have supplied.

The candidate must not be younger than eighteen years, nor older than thirty-five; and if under twenty-one, he must furnish evidence that he is about to enter the service by consent of his parents or guardians.

If, however, the applicant has been in the army before, he may be received although he is over thirty-five years. If he re-enlists before two months have expired, he receives $2 50 extra pay per month, the extra pay dating back two months. If he intends to enter the ranks as a musician, he may be younger than eighteen years.

It is the general opinion of army surgeons that eighteen years is too young. The various organs of the body are not at this period of life completely developed, and such persons are often incapable of that endurance which is so necessary to a complete soldier. It is also often impossible to foresee what will be the character of the constitution when the growth and development are completed. Sir George Ballingall says: "Upon a full consideration of all the circumstances, I think we may state that the most eligible period of life for enlistment is from twenty to twenty-five years of age;" and perhaps it would serve the interests of the government equally well if young men were never admitted until they were fully of age, since the department would thus be saved the heavy expense incident to the enrolment of minors whose parents or guardians subsequently obtain their release.

The opinion of that great general, Napoleon, of the relative value of boys and men as soldiers, may be inferred from his communication to the Senate after the battle of Leipsic, and when some of its members had shown a reluctance to accede to his demands. "Shame on you," said the Emperor, "I demand a levy of 300,000 men. But I must have grown men; boys serve only to encumber the hospitals and roadsides."

As pertinent to this subject it may be remarked, also, that in the naval service, where enlistments are made at a very early period of life, examples of extreme longevity are much more rare than in the army.

The regulations relating to height have varied in different countries and in different periods, and seem to have been made generally with reference to the exigencies of the service. At present the minimum for the British regular service is five feet five and a half inches, and in the Anglo-Indian army it is five feet six inches. Formerly the British regulations demanded five feet six and a half for the infantry, and five feet seven for the cavalry. In the French army the present minimum is five feet one inch and nearly one half, but men are not unfrequently enlisted who are only five feet one inch.

In our service the standard has been frequently changed. By an Act of Congress in 1790 it was fixed at five feet six inches; but in 1796 this law was repealed and the matter left subject to the regulations of the Army Board. During the war with Mexico, the regulations demanded only five feet three inches; but by the regulations of 1854 it was fixed at five feet four and a half inches, and such is the requirement at the present time.

The experience afforded by the Crimean war, where the English soldiers labored side and side, in the trenches, upon marches, and in the assault, prove conclusively that the additional stature of the English troops gave them no advantage over the French. Now that battles are no longer decided so much by weight of arm as by strategy, promptness of action, rapidity of movement and precision of aim—length of limb and even power of muscle are not so essential. What is needed now in the soldier is activity and endurance, and these are by no means the peculiar attributes of size or even of simple muscular strength. A man of short stature will frequently endure a long and forced march better than a tall man; and we have seen professed pugilists who would lose their breath, and be placed completely *hors de combat*, by a rapid walk up a moderate acclivity.

Weight.—We do not think any man ought to be accepted who weighs over 200 or 220 lbs., and who is at the same time below 6 feet in height; nor, on the other hand, ought he to be received if he is too slight or puny, with a weight of less than 100 lbs. 'Perhaps on an average it may be stated that the best soldiers are composed of men who weigh from 135 to 150 lbs.

Striking Deformity.—The soldier ought to have something like proportion and harmony in the different portions of his body; not so much for the reason that he will present a more soldier-like appearance, and is likely to have more self-respect, but because marked deviations from the usual law of nature generally imply physical infirmity. A head large or small, out of proportion to the body; arms or legs either too long or too short; very crooked legs, a deformed chest, or any other deformity sufficiently unusual to excite attention and remark, indicate in general the early existence of some constitutional malady which, although it may have ceased to progress, great exposure or fatigue may awaken into a fatal activity.

Intemperance.—Habitual intemperance is a sufficient ground for rejection, not only because the soldier will be tempted on every possible opportunity to drink, but especially because the constitution of such a man is in all probability seriously impaired, if not irretrievably ruined. Moreover, says Dr. Tripler, "first in a mutiny and last in a battle, the intemperate soldier is, at once, an example of insubordination, and a nuisance to his comrades."

It is a positive rule of the service not to accept of a man who is at the time of the examination intoxicated; but if he repeats his application when he is sober, or if he only shows signs of a recent debauch, it will then be necessary to ascertain whether his intoxication was accidental, or whether he is habitually an intemperate drinker. The man who has been accidentally betrayed into intoxication may look pale, his eyes heavy and somewhat reddened; but the habitual drunkard has, in most cases, his face and nose studded with pimples, his lids are red and thickened, his eyes blood-shot and watery, his hands tremble, and his tongue refuses to articulate distinctly; his breath has a peculiar odor, and the whole muscular system is frequently in a condition of atrophy. Especially is this the case with the muscles of the lower extremities.

Moral Character.—It is necessary also to the preservation of discipline, that the recruit should not be a bad man, or a thorough villain. Convicted felons, men who have suffered imprisonment in jails or state prisons for criminal offences, deserters, and professional fighters, are not proper men to be received. They are troublesome, refractory, and soon poison the minds of others.

Having made these preliminary inquiries and examinations, we are now prepared to enter into a more minute investigation of the applicant's condition. For this purpose, he ought to be washed and stripped, and we should commence the examination at the head, in order that we may proceed systematically and overlook nothing.

Baldness, when not excessive, cannot be regarded as a disqualifying circumstance, but when a large portion of the scalp is exposed in a person under thirty-five years of age, it may lead to a suspicion that the subject is laboring under secondary or tertiary syphilis, or that he is suffering from some other grave constitutional malady; and besides, the soldier who is bald finds it inconvenient to keep upon his head the military cap, and when uncovered he is peculiarly exposed to the intense heat of the sun in summer, and to the cold of winter.

Chronic eruptive affections of the scalp, of whatever character, if extensive, ought to be regarded as disqualifying conditions. Their cure is likely to prove troublesome; they exact on the part of the man himself greater care and time for cleanliness, and it is not certain but that they may be conveyed to others.

A very large or very small head, as we have already intimated, implies imperfect development or hypertrophy, neither of which is consistent with a perfect constitution.

Tumors of the Scalp. One, or even two or three small encysted tumors upon the scalp could scarcely be regarded as of sufficient importance to demand a rejection, unless they happened to be situated just where the cap would press upon and inflame them. They are not likely to become sources of trouble unless an attempt is made to remove them. Tumors of almost any other kind, even fatty tumors, as they are apt to attain a great size, are causes for rejection.

Old wounds of the scalp ought to invite an inquiry into the cause, and especially with a view to ascertain whether the skull has been broken, or any cerebral symptoms followed the accident. We have known cases in which, after severe blows upon the scalp, although, so far as could be ascertained, no fracture had taken place, yet epilepsy has, after the lapse of many years, supervened.

We ought certainly to reject every applicant whose skull has been broken at any period of life.

If the fracture was limited in extent and no fragments were ever removed, even though the depression was very slight, our own experience shows that epilepsy is very likely to supervene at some period of life. And if the fracture was extensive, and fragments of bone have been removed, the subject is still liable to cephalic pains and congestions from any unusual exertion, and he is wholly unfit for the duties of a soldier.

Defects in hearing, when permanent and incurable, render the applicant unfit for admission to the ranks, since he is liable to misunderstand the orders. If, however, it is temporary, depending upon a cold, which has swollen the tonsils or the mucous membrane of the mouth, and produced an occlusion of the eustachian tubes, or when it depends solely upon wax or some foreign body in the ear, the applicant may be admitted whenever the cure is accomplished, or even before, if the surgeon feels quite certain as to the cause of the deafness.

Obliteration of the auditory canal, chronic eczema of the canal, a discharge of matter, malformation, or loss of a portion of the external ear, generally disqualify.

Sight. We may first examine the condition of the lids, brows, and of the lacrymal apparatus, since it is no more important that the sight should be perfect, than that the means of preservation should be complete.

A total absence of the eye-brows, equally with baldness

of the head, implies generally the existence of a cachexy, or constitutional vice; moreover, the eye has lost in consequence one of its most important means of protection. The eyebrows are black and long in the natives of tropical climates, and all persons have more or less the power of corrugating and lowering the brow in order to exclude the too intense and direct rays of the sun. They serve, also, by their peculiar arrangement, the superciliæ being imbricated and inclined downwards and outwards, to direct the perspiration upon the temples, and thus to protect the eye from those acrid salts which accompany this secretion.

Eyelashes. Absence of the eyelashes also, is generally accompanied with chronic tarsal ophthalmia, or with trichiasis, and is a sufficient ground for rejection.

Chronic tarsal ophthalmia, being either, in general, a mark of intemperance or of a scrofulous diathesis, is a disqualifying circumstance. The upper and lower lids ought to be everted and examined carefully, and the position of the ciliæ upon the margins of the lids should be noted.

Eversion or inversion of the lids disqualifies.

Ptosis, whether congenital, from paralysis, or as a result of chronic inflammation, is a cause for rejection.

The existence of small encysted tumors, which are very common upon the upper lid, and seldom attain a greater size than a pea, need not constitute an objection.

Obstructions of the lacrymal ducts, at whatever point, or from whatever cause, are liable to recur or to continue; and since such obstructions occasion great annoyance, and even at length lead to sensible impairment of vision, they ought to be regarded as causes for rejection.

A pterygium, unless it is very small and not progressive, ought to occasion rejection. Its tendency to encroach more and more upon the cornea until it reaches the centre, is very great; nor is it always a very curable affection, even when subjected to the knife.

Strabismus, in either eye, or in any direction, ought to be a cause for rejection. The strabismic eye is, in a great majority of cases, myopic, and such persons are very apt to see objects double.

In the Manual the conclusion is reached that strabismus of the right eye disqualifies for any service; but if it is only in the left eye, the subject is not disqualified for infantry or artillery service, but only for cavalry. In this opinion we can scarcely agree with the author of the Manual, or with the author of the "Aide-Memoire," to whom reference is made as sustaining this view.

The fact is, that strabismics are in general not so vigorous as others; their vision is occasionally double, the vision of one eye being usually myopic; the strabismic eye wearies under long use, and is more prone to inflame. These statements will be found very well established in a monograph upon strabismus, with a reference to a large number of cases, which we published in 1842.

Ulcerations of the cornea: hernia iridis: staphyloma: are sufficient causes for rejection.

Opacity of the cornea, if the result of recent inflammation, however limited in extent, is a sufficient cause for rejection; since it is not certain but that it will increase, and the inflammation having only recently disappeared it is very liable to return.

If the opacity is ancient and not extensive, and does not interfere with correct vision, it may not be a sufficient cause for rejection.

Irregularity of the pupil, such as to affect vision; adhesion of the pupil, are causes for rejection.

Cataract, glaucoma, amaurosis, whether in one or both eyes, we need scarcely say, demand rejection; so also, hydrophthalmia, exophthalmia, and vascillitans bulbi.

Myopia, if considerable, is a sufficient cause for rejection.

Presbyopia is not a cause for rejection unless it is very decided.

Loss of the nose usually implies in this country, the prior existence of a syphilitic taint. But from whatever cause it may be wanting, the disfigurement is such as to render the subject liable to cruel jests, and to be an object of disgust to his companions.

Obstructions of the nose, such as to impede free respiration through the nasal passages, whether from polypi, ozœna, morbid thickening of the mucous membrane, or from any other cause whatever, provided always these causes are known to be chronic or incurable, are disqualifying conditions.

Hare-lip, or any striking deformity of the mouth, from burns, wounds, or disease, disqualifies.

The loss of many teeth, or if they are generally unsound. The teeth are needful not only for mastication of tough salt meat, and "hard tack," but also for biting off the cartridge.

Disease or mutilation of the tongue is a disqualification. So also is stammering, if it exist in any considerable degree.

Chronic enlargement of the tonsils is generally a sign of a scrofulous diathesis.

A large goitre, interfering with respiration, or such as prevents the wearing a stock comfortably; enlargement of the submaxillary, sublingual, or parotid glands, or of several of the absorbent glands of the neck; the existence of old cicatrices occasioned by suppuration of these glands, ought to disqualify.

Malformation of the chest, sufficient to embarrass respiration. If the chest is narrow in its transverse diameter, and exceedingly prominent in front, a "chicken breast," as it is called, it is not probable that the man will endure long marches well; especially if at the same time the shoulder-blades stand off from the back of the chest ("winged shoulder-blades"), and are imperfectly covered with muscles. These men may give no positive sign of lesions of the lungs, and yet all experience shows that they are more than others predisposed to tubercular and other affections of the thoracic viscera.

A flattening of one side of the chest from chronic pleurisy; organic and even serious functional diseases of the heart, forbid the acceptance of a recruit.

Asthma is usually spasmodic, occurring only at intervals, and it is possible therefore for an applicant to impose upon the recruiting officer, by presenting himself when the paroxysm is off. But if it has existed long, it is probable that such permanent lesions of the heart and respiratory organs will be present as will determine the fact of unsoundness independently of the asthma.

Enlargement of the abdominal viscera, whether of the liver, spleen, or of any other organ; ascites or tympanitis, are disqualifying diseases.

The fact that the person is very subject to diarrhœa or to dysentery, or even to violent attacks of colic, is sometimes a ground for rejection.

Complete absence of the penis; epispadias, hypospadias, at or beyond the middle of the penis; stricture of the penis, a perineal fistula, incontinence of urine, as causing inconvenience in urination; castration, complete atrophy or great hypertrophy of the testicles, indicating some constitutional malady, or rendering the person liable to suffer from slight causes in these organs; all enlargements of the testicles, or of the seminal ducts, or distensions of the tunica vaginalis; the existence of chronic eczema in these parts, should occasion rejection.

If the testicles have never descended, or having descended, may be occasionally retracted partly or entirely within the abdomen, the person is more liable to a hernia.

Varicocele. Dr. Tripler says, that "out of 5,000 rejections in our service, 877 were for varicose veins and varicocele." He properly adds, "if men are to be rejected for this affection indiscriminately, our rendezvous might almost as well be closed."

The truth is, that a moderate varicocele seldom is anything more than a source of inconvenience, and one which the wearing of an ordinary suspensory bandage will usually relieve. It is not, therefore, without some qualifications, a ground for rejection.

We would say, if the varicocele is of the size of a butternut; if it is very painful, as we have in two or three instances known it to be; if it is attended with much emaciation of the corresponding testicle, or with other varices in other portions of the body, we would regard it as a ground for rejection.

Prolapsus ani, stricture of the rectum, fistula in ano, we need not say, are positive disqualifications. We would ourselves say the same of hæmorrhoids, whether external or internal, so long as they remain uncured; but Dr. Tripler remarks that this is a very common affection, and "to exclude all men so affected without regard to extent or degree, would be equally unjust to the recruit and to the service."

In the British Regulations, hæmorrhoids are said to disqualify "when they exist to such a degree as will immediately, or in all probability may at no distant period, impair a man's efficiency."

Dr. Tripler asks how are we to determine whether they are likely hereafter to disqualify? If internal, we cannot, unless we see them bleeding or discharging pus; but if external, he says by examination and by the testimony of the man himself; yet we have often seen cases of simple external piles, uninflamed, which occasioned no inconvenience until the man has mounted a horse, or has had an attack of diarrhœa or of constipation, and then they have at once become very troublesome.

Would it not be a better rule in all these cases to direct the applicant to submit to a very simple operation for their cure, namely, excision, and to return to the rendezvous when the cure is completed?

Hernia. The existence of any form or degree of abdominal hernia ought to be regarded as sufficient cause for rejection.

It is a question, however, whether large abdominal rings can be regarded as conditions predisposing to hernia. It will be observed that the external abdominal ring varies greatly in size in different persons who never have had a hernia. We have noticed this both in the dissecting room and in examination of living persons. It is only a few days since that we were consulted by a young man who said he had been rejected as an applicant for the office of policeman in the City of New York, on the ground that the external rings were large. We found them sufficiently large to admit freely the forefinger, and we could carry this finger up to the internal ring. There was no hernia in the canal, and the internal ring was close and firm.

This man had been a sailor during the last seven or eight years, doing duty before the mast. He was a strong, muscular man, and we cannot think he was likely to have a hernia. Indeed, it is not so much the condition of the external ring as of the internal which disposes to rupture.

If, however, the person has an oblong swelling in the situation of the canal, it is probable that an internal hernia already exists, and it may be a sufficient cause for rejection.

In examining the recruit to ascertain the existence of a rupture, the finger should be introduced into the external ring. This is best done by placing the point of the finger at first low down upon the scrotum and carrying it up, as it were, through the scrotum. By this method the finger enters easily the inguinal canal, while if it is applied directly from over the ring it is always more difficult to feel and often impossible to enter the ring. The subject must be then directed to cough while the finger of the surgeon is in this position, and while the hands of the subject are extended and clasped over the head.

Spinal distortions, of whatever character, if seen to be the result of disease, such as rachitis in early life, or of caries (Pott's disease), or of muscular weakness, indicated by a lateral curvature, ought to cause rejection. Even persons who are exceedingly round-shouldered are not usually proper subjects for active military service. They are not likely to have the same thoracic capacity; and they are, especially when loaded with their knapsacks, very unsoldierly men for a line.

We must next proceed to examine the condition of the extremities, and for this purpose the man will be instructed to walk, run, jump, hop, kneel, extend and flex his arms, &c. &c. It is the opinion of Jackson that "a full grown person who is not capable of marching at the rate of four miles in the hour, with firelock and knapsack, is not eligible for a soldier destined for the field service. If his wind fail in walking briskly up hill, or if his joints be weak, so that he does not move with speed and safety over broken grounds, it would be unwise to enrol him on the lists of an active army." He therefore thinks that it would "be proper that every person who enters the army should be brought to trial in walking, running, leaping, climbing hills, and traversing irregularly broken grounds." Dr. Tripler, who approves of this rigid course of inspection, especially since the introduction into our service of the severe drill of the *chasseur-à-pied*, nevertheless thinks that in the places where these inspections are generally made such tests of capacity are impossible.

The custom of recruiting officers in this country is to exercise and display the points of the recruit somewhat in the following manner.

He is first walked around the room on a rapid gait, then he is directed to run, then hop a short distance first on one leg and then on the other. He is then halted and set up in the position of a soldier under arms, with the knees about one inch apart, and while in this position he may be examined again in front and in rear. He is then directed to extend his arms at a right angle with his body, touch the shoulder with the fingers, place the backs of his hands together above his head, flex and extend his arms, rotate the forearm, flex and extend the wrist and each finger and thumb. The recruit should be directed to stand first upon one foot, and then upon the other, moving the ankle joint while standing upon the floor; he should kneel, first upon one knee and then upon the other, and subsequently upon both, being made to rise each time without touching his hands to the floor.

The surgeon ought to examine carefully with his hand every part of the upper and lower extremities.

A fracture of the clavicle anywhere through the middle third, united with a manifest overlapping, disqualifies, not by diminishing the strength of the limb, but by rendering it inconvenient to wear the knapsack strap. If, however, the fracture has been at any other point, and it is united, it ought not to disqualify.

A dislocation, or partial dislocation of the clavicle at either end, if unreduced, actually impairs the strength of the arm; especially in holding a weight at a right angle with the body, or in lifting a weight above the shoulders.

Fractures of the shaft of the humerus, even though badly united, do not, after a year or two, generally maim the arm; but if they are in the vicinity of the joints, they often produce more or less anchylosis, and of course, in such a case, disqualify.

After a dislocation, also, either of the shoulder or elbow, there may exist anchylosis or atrophy, but it is by no means constant.

Fractures of the radius and ulna do not necessarily maim, even if badly united, yet they are more likely to do so than fractures of the humerus.

Fractures of fingers, and of other bones of the hand, often leave no maiming.

A dislocated finger, however, is pretty certain to be followed by some anchylosis.

We ought to ascertain that there are no ganglions about the wrist.

Webbed fingers, split fingers, loss of either phalanx of the thumb or forefinger of the right hand, loss of two or more phalanges of either finger of the right hand, loss of either thumb, loss of any two fingers of either hand, mutilation of all the last phalanges of either hand, complete anchylosis of any finger, but especially of the forefinger of the right hand, are absolute disqualifications.

Fractures of the neck of the femur always cause lameness.

Fractures of the shaft, in adults, usually unite with overlapping, but unless this is sufficient to make the man limp, it ought not to disqualify.

Fractures of the patella probably always render the person less able to endure long marches. So also all fractures involving the knee-joint.

Dislocations at either end of the femur may cause stiffness, but if reduced, especially in the case of the hip-joint, no lameness may follow.

Fractures of the leg, also, in general cause lameness, or weakness; but not so generally as in case of the femur, unless the fracture be at the lower end, involving the joint, or it be accompanied with a dislocation.

We think a complete luxation of the ankle, or a fracture of any of the bones of the tarsus, always produces some weakness in the foot.

The surgeon should carefully examine and compare the two knees. If swollen, or enlarged, or very much bent in, so as to render the man "knock-kneed," he should be rejected. The existence of a bursa at this point should also cause his rejection.

Varicose veins, if considerable, or if attended with œdema, or ulcerations, or dark spots, are causes for rejection.

"Ulcerations demanding rejection are those combined with great loss of substance; with atrophy of the limb; with general constitutional disorder, or with varicose veins."

Club-feet positively disqualify.

Splay-feet, or those in which the natural arches are

almost completely lost, do not necessarily disqualify. It is very common to find this form of foot among the laboring people, especially upon the continent of Europe. These men may, after a little, become very good soldiers.

But valgus absolutely disqualifies. In these cases the arches are not only lost, but the muscles behind the malleolus internus being preternaturally weak, as well as the ligaments on this side elongated, the ankle-joint falls inwards, as the knees do in cases of knock-knee, so that the inner border of the os naviculare actually touches the ground. Such persons generally turn the toes very much out, and walk with the inner side of the foot presenting forwards.

Loss of a great toe; loss of any two toes of the same foot; webbed toes; double toes; the great toe crossing the second very much, so as to render the metatarso-phalangeal articulation very prominent; much overriding of all the toes; permanent retraction of the last phalanx, so that the free border of the nail touches the ground; ingrowing and ulceration of the nails, are all actual disqualifications.

Epilepsy, if it has occurred within five years; chorea; paralysis of any member; scrofula; constitutional syphilis, disqualify for the military service.

The Manual would not consider the "primitive accidents of syphilis" as an insuperable ground for rejection; but we cannot agree with the author in this opinion.

Itch, and chronic incurable diseases of the skin, of a constitutional or specific character, &c., are disqualifying maladies.

General feebleness of constitution, with constitutions like women; brands for desertion or for drunkenness, disqualify.

MODE OF EXAMINING A RECRUIT.

COPIED FROM THE MANUAL.

"The room in which this examination is conducted should be well lighted and large enough to admit of the men being walked about freely, that every organ concerned in locomotion may be subjected to inspection. For obvious reasons, none others than they whose presence is absolutely required, should be admitted to the room.

"The person of the recruit should be washed *clean* before he is presented to the surgeon for inspection. It is impossible for the medical officer to ascertain the existence of certain defects that *absolutely disqualify*, when concealed, as they effectually may be and sometimes are, by incrustations of filth a month old.

"We have remarked that certain defects can be ascertained only by questioning the man himself, and that, in order to avoid all subsequent evasions, the answers to these questions should be recorded on the spot. We shall now suggest a method of effecting this object, as well as of making it sure that no important part shall escape inspection through any slip of the memory.

"The following printed form is to be furnished upon which the observations of the inspecting surgeon are to be recorded as they are made.

Recruit A. B.
Age Years,
Occupation,
Born in
Presented by

1. Have you ever been sick? When and of what diseases?
2. Have you any disease now? (Such as diarrhœa, cough, and the like.)
3. Have you ever had fits?

4. Have you ever received an injury or wound upon the head?

5. Have you ever had a fracture, a dislocation, or a sprain?

6. Are you in the habit of drinking? or, have you ever had the "horrors?"

7. Are you subject to the piles?

8. Have you any difficulty in urinating?

9. Have you been vaccinated? or, had the small-pox?

Head.
Ears.
Face.
Eyes and appendages.
Nose.
Organs of mastication and voice.
Neck.
Chest.
Abdomen.
Genital and urinary organs.
Vertebral column.
Superior extremities.
Inferior extremities.

REMARKS.

(Approved or rejected as the case may be.)
Date,
Rendezvous.

Inspecting Surgeon.

"The questions should be asked and the man's answers recorded before he is stripped.

"He is then to be divested of *all* his clothing and the examination proceeded with systematically, in the order of regions as indicated in the 'Form.'

"The surgeon is to note every peculiarity or deviation from the normal standard in each particular region. For example—If the man has received at any time a blow upon the head, with a resulting cicatrix, or slight depression, let it be noted thus—'Cicatrix and slight depression upon the right parietal protuberance.'

"Scars upon any part of the person should be noted, and the cause assigned by the man, recorded. It is not uncommon to find marks of free cupping upon the chests of Germans, without their being any indication of disease. These, however, should be noted.

"If, upon inspection, the man be found to have a circocele, though not sufficient to disqualify, let it be noted under the proper head; and so of hæmorrhoids, or any other affection. The vaccine scar and its position should be noted, and whether vaccination has been practised at the rendezvous or depôt.

"Under the head of 'Remarks,' constitutional syphilis, or other cachexiæ, will find a place. If an interpreter is required during the inspection, that fact should be recorded. Men sometimes speak English very well when first examined, who, from after considerations, are entirely ignorant of the language when re-examined, and sometimes succeed in obtaining a discharge in this way.

"By this means an accurate description of the whole person is obtained, sufficient to settle questions of identity, should such be subsequently raised; and if there be any defects about which a difference of opinion may exist, the fact that such defects were not overlooked by the first inspecting surgeon, will be apparent.

"It will frequently happen that an 'absolute disqualification' will be discovered before completing the examination. Such a defect may be detected at any stage of the inspection. In such cases it will of course be unnecessary to proceed any further.

"The above form, when filled up, should be sent with the recruit to the depôt, where he is to be finally inspected, and thence transmitted to the regiment to which he may be assigned.

"Defects discovered at the depôt upon re-inspection should be endorsed upon the form, and signed by the surgeon; in case of rejection the document thus completed, should be transmitted with the proceedings of the board of inspection to the headquarters of the Army."

REGULATIONS FOR THE EXAMINATION OF RECRUITS IN THE UNITED STATES NAVY.

The following are the rules adopted for the examination of recruits in the United States Navy, as given in the "Instructions for the Government of the Medical Officers of the Navy of the United States," published at Washington in 1857.

Surgeons of rendezvous, or on recruiting service, will be particularly attentive in the examination of recruits. They will cause each recruit to be stripped of all his clothes, to move about, exercise his limbs in their presence, in order to ascertain whether he has free use of them; that his chest is ample; that his hearing, vision, and speech are good; that he has no tumors, ulcerated or extensively cicatrized legs, rupture, chronic cutaneous affection, or other disorder or infirmity, mental or physical, which may render him unfit for the active duties of the navy.

They will ascertain, as far as practicable, whether the recruit be subject to convulsions of any kind, or has received any contusion or wounds of the head which may produce occasional insanity. With any of these defects, the man will be rejected.

Attention will also be paid as to whether or not the recruit exhibit satisfactory evidence of vaccination or palpable exemption from variola, that the unprotected may be immediately vaccinated by the surgeon of the vessel to which the recruit may be transferred.

No person will be received into the service without having previously undergone the necessary inspection; nor will pensioners from the Naval Asylum be allowed to enter the general service.

If, however, persons should be entered for particular ratings with physical defects, which, in the opinion of the surgeon and commander of the station, may not disqualify them for the duties of such rate, these defects are *to be fully described* and reported by the surgeon to this Bureau, to prevent any subsequent claim for pension on account of such injuries and defects.

CHAPTER III.

GENERAL HYGIENE OF TROOPS.

SECTION I.—DIET. The food supplied to soldiers, whether in the field or in barracks, ought to be wholesome and abundant. We scarcely need to say that we do not demand for the army a luxurious diet; but only that those who serve their country faithfully, should, whenever it is possible, have enough food to satisfy all reasonable wants; and that, however coarse and plain it may be, it should be nutritious.

As to a luxurious mode of living, whether we consider it in its relations to the soldiers or to the officers, no one entertains a doubt of its pernicious effects. It has proved the destruction of many fine armies which were invincible to all other enemies.

Great military chieftains, who have led their armies to conquest, have been nearly always men of frugal habits and unaccustomed to a sumptuous fare. Says Jackson, "it is reported that General Wolfe, who was perhaps the most perfect soldier of the age in which he lived, never gave an elegant, and rarely an eatable dinner to persons of the *haut gout.* General Wolfe's table was said to be an epitome of a Spartan mess-room—no one rose from it without having been furnished with the opportunity of carrying away a military lesson; and few left it without feeling an accession of military importance communicated to the mind by the impressive influence of a hero's spirit."

As to the particular articles of diet, no special rules can be established, since these must depend upon the season of the year, the nature of the country through which the troops are to pass, the character of the diseases to which they will be most exposed, and upon the ability of the commissary to meet the demands made upon him.

In general it is impossible to keep troops constantly supplied with fresh meat and fresh vegetables, especially when they are upon long marches; yet it is always desirable, at least in this country, that they should have both in a certain proportion. Where this is impracticable, the army must be furnished with salted or dried meats, dried vegetables and fruit, and with hard bread, as the next best alternatives. The salted meats are generally either beef or pork. The dried ("desiccated") meats, vegetables, and fruits, are now prepared at home, as well as in France, and in other foreign countries; and they are usually supplied to the army of the United States whenever it is ordered upon distant expeditions. They may be obtained at the office of Messrs. Copland and Shutes, No. 56 South Street, New York. These gentlemen have on hand constantly about eighteen varieties of desiccated vegetables and fruits, including potatoes, onions, cabbage, tomatoes, carrots, turnips, string-beans, green peas, asparagus, apples, etc. They prepare also in the same manner a "beef soup," of which one half is composed of desiccated meat, and the other half of eight different vegetables; one ounce of this produces about one quart of most excellent soup, as we can ourselves attest. Their "beef stew," composed of beef, potatoes, and onions, is equally palatable.

When we consider the compactness—dried and compressed, as they are, under heavy hydraulic pressure—the lightness, the imperishable nature, of these articles, we must understand their value as army supplies, at all seasons of the year; but it is especially when troops are sent into the northwestern territories, and beyond the reach of winter supplies, that they are furnished usually with extra quantities of desiccated vegetables and fruits, as an important means of protection against scurvy.

Concentrated milk, prepared eggs, prepared extract of coffee, are furnished in the most compact form by the same gentlemen. Solidified milk may be found at 73 Liberty Street, New York.

Bread is with all civilized nations an important article of diet, and it is especially so in grain-growing countries like our own. It is necessary, therefore, that the supplies of this article should be ample in quantity, and suitable in quality. Dr. Mann, in his "Medical Sketches," enumerates among the active causes which led to the production of disease among the troops along the Niagara frontier during the campaign of 1812, "bad bread." "It was notorious," he remarks, "that the bread on the Niagara was made of damaged flour; such as was either not nutritious, or absolutely deleterious. It was believed, also, that the flour contained, in some instances, an earthy substance, and that this adulterating substance was plaster of Paris."

In relation to alcoholic liquors as a part of the rations to soldiers, Dr. Mann, whose opinions, from their eminently practical nature, we are happy always to quote, speaks as follows: "My opinion long has been, that ardent spirits are an unnecessary part of a ration. This allowance, as a part of a ration, is not, however, the evil which demands a remedy. It is the abuse of spirits. Sutlers unrestrained, as they frequently are, destroy more lives by these liquors, than are lost by other causes to which soldiers are exposed; and, so long as ardent spirits are permitted to be publicly sold in the vicinity of a cantonment, these evils cannot be remedied by any restrictions under which sutlers may be placed. A soldier habitually intemperate, is always industrious to procure the means of indulging his appetite. All his cunning and every artifice are put into requisition to obtain the inebriating draught. Reputation, honor, health, and even life, are sacrificed to his gratification.

"Examples may be furnished to demonstrate that ardent spirits are a useless part of a soldier's ration. At those periods, during the revolutionary war, when the army received no pay for their services, and possessed not the means to procure spirits, it was healthy. The 4th Massachusetts regiment at that eventful period, of which I was the surgeon, lost in three years, by sickness, not more than five or six men. It was at a time when the army was destitute of money. During the winter of '79-'80, there was only one occurrence of fever in the regiment, and that was a pneumonia of a mild form. It was observable in the last war, from December, 1814, to April, 1815, the soldiers at Plattsburgh were not attacked with fevers as they had been the preceding winters. The troops, during this period, were not paid; a fortunate circumstance to the army, arising from a want of funds. This embarrassment, which was considered a national calamity, proved a blessing to the soldier. When he is found poor in money, it is always the case that he abounds in health. A fact worth recording!"

It is now several years since, mainly through the recommendations of Gen. Cass, while Secretary of War, the whiskey rations were stopped in the United States Army, and rations of coffee and sugar substituted. Sutlers are expressly forbidden to keep it among their stores; yet it is found impossible, except when stationed out of the reach of civilization, to prevent the soldiers from obtaining it occasionally, or some equally pernicious substitute.

Assistant Surgeon Bartholomew, in his report to the Surgeon-General, March, 1859, speaking of the condition of the troops stationed at Fort Bridger, Utah Territory, remarks: "A vile concoction, known as whiskey, has been from time to time surreptitiously sold to the troops, notwithstanding prohibitory orders from the commanding officer. Manufactured by traders, from alcohol, tobacco, and other narcotics, this liquor has in one instance produced an immediately fatal effect, and more or less alarming symptoms in various instances."

In Mexico many of our soldiers were made sick, and not a few died in consequence of having drunk the pulque, a stimulating drink obtained from the Agave Americana, a species of cactus which grows abundantly in that country.

Wellington had his rations invariably delivered to the soldiers daily, unless the circumstances were such as to render this impossible, for the reason that he found that men would eat up or waste in a single day what was intended for two or three, trusting to chance, to forays, or to opportunities for purchase, to supply themselves until the rations were distributed again.

We think it necessary that soldiers should have three meals per day; especially is this deemed necessary for soldiers who are American citizens, and who have become accustomed to the habits of our own people in this respect. These meals may consist in general of a light breakfast of bread and coffee, taken always before the morning parade, or the march—a substantial dinner of meat and vegetables at midday, and a pretty substantial supper at the close of the day.

Soldiers should be encouraged to mess; and one of the

first things they need to learn is how to cook. The art of cookery is as important to the soldier as the art of defence: and especially as the one is in requisition daily, while the other is in demand only at long intervals.

By dividing the men into squads of three or five, and by detailing alternately one of the men to prepare the meals by an established order of fatigue, a sort of emulation will be encouraged to excel, while each will learn from observing the ingenious expedients of the other, and very soon they will all acquire a tolerable degree of excellence. The culinary art is simple, and with any man of common intelligence easily acquired. Salted meats should be well soaked before they are cooked, and soups should be made from the meats by the addition of such vegetables and condiments as may be at hand in the commissary's stores, or as can be obtained in the adjacent fields—" C'est la soupe qui fait le soldat." The meat may be afterwards placed in the haversack, and eaten cold at the next meal or on the march, if needed; but whether meats are boiled or roasted, it is a fundamental rule to boil slowly, and roast quickly.

Sudden changes, even from a bad to a better diet, have not unfrequently proved disastrous to troops. During the Mexican war, most of the men who were brought down to Vera Cruz from the Rio Grande, had to march over the country by the way of Tampico, having only salted meat, and that chiefly pork, with hard bread and beans. Those who went in transports fared no better. Soon after leaving Vera Cruz, however, the soldiers fell in with large droves of cattle, which they slaughtered, and eat of the fresh meat freely. In consequence of this, diarrhœa and dysentery began to prevail, and before they reached Cerro Gordo the army was already in a bad condition from this cause. At Jalapa, where great numbers of the sick and wounded were crowded into a cold stone church, a great many died. Perote also proved equally fatal to the troops, although it was accounted one of the most healthy situations in Mexico. The soldiers died not only of dysentery in great numbers, but, in consequence of the prevalence of bowel affections, nearly all the wounded did badly. The wounds did not generally become gangrenous, but they refused to heal, and the patients sank from the continued and exhausting suppuration.

SECTION II.—"CLEANLINESS is the life of an army, while filth and dirt are among its disease-generating causes. The observance of cleanliness in domestic life is of the highest importance to secure the body in health. It is no less valuable as a means of supporting the strength and efficient force of an army in actual service. Filth and dirt become more active destroyers of life when they co-operate with pestilential states of atmosphere, or insalubrious gases, the production of unhealthy climates, or noxious situations. Cleanliness should be enforced upon soldiers with most rigid laws. The code under the Jewish dispensation, enforcing ablutions and purifications, was obeyed as a religious rite: it has been quoted as a system well adapted to a camp. It has been observed that those regiments which have been subjected to rigid discipline, and where cleanliness has been strongly enforced, have enjoyed higher states of health than those who have been inattentive to this duty. * * * * * There was one regiment on the frontiers, which at one time counted nine hundred strong, but was reduced by a total want of good police to less than two hundred fit for duty in the course of two months. This regiment, in its appearance, was at that time dirty in the extreme. To save the remains, if possible, General Dearborn found it necessary to place it under the command of Colonel Miller (now General) by annexing it to his regiment. At one period more than three hundred and forty of this regiment were in hospitals; in addition to these, a large number were reported sick in camp. At the close of the war, this regiment had established a high reputation. Its good discipline and bravery were excelled by none.

"The regiments of heavy and light artillery suffered less by disease during the war, than any other regiments on the northern frontiers. It is unnecessary to observe, these regiments are always subject to correct discipline; and their better health may be much imputed to cleanliness. Their quarters and encampments were generally in the best state; the men were, mostly, neat and clean in their dress and appearance."

To these judicious remarks and observations of Dr. Mann nothing needs to be added. We cannot omit, however, to call attention to a letter of Dr. Griscom, of New York, published in the *Amer. Journ. of Med. Science*, May, 1833, describing the terrible mortality which prevailed on board the ship Sybilla, during her passage from Holland to this port, and which he ascribes solely to "their horribly filthy condition." The whole number of emigrants who left Holland was one hundred and thirty-two, of whom ninety-four perished on the voyage.

SECTION III.—DRESS. This is a matter having intimate relations to general hygiene. Yet, we regret to say that in the selection of the materials, and in the construction of a soldier's dress, there is too often more regard paid to the general effect, than to the comfort and health of the wearer. No doubt something must be conceded to the exterior appearance of troops; there needs to be a proportion and harmony, and, perhaps, a certain amount of "millinery," in order to the preservation of a proper military effect; but we think that this never need to interfere with the quality, form, or abundant and suitable supply of clothing.

The dress ought to be suited to the climate, season, and to the character or nature of the expedition in which the troops are to be employed. In this climate, during most of the season, the general object of dress is to protect the surface of the body from cold; and that it may not at the same time interfere with perfect freedom of motion, it needs to be warm, light, and free.

The cap should be light, and with ample space within the crown for ventilation. We have seen recently some regiments of Zouaves furnished with tight fitting skull-caps, which afford neither protection against the cold nor the direct rays of the sun; and, when we consider that these regiments are composed of raw recruits, men mostly accustomed to wear hats or high-topped caps, and that they have been submitted immediately after enlistment to "cropping," by which they are deprived of the ordinary protection of the hair, we must see that they will suffer greatly in a warm climate, and during the intense heats of summer. The cap ought to be at the same time a protection against the extreme vicissitudes of heat and cold, against rain and snow; and, moreover, it may be firm enough to become a partial defence against the stroke of an enemy's sabre. In no case ought the front piece or visor to be omitted. Soldiers without this important protection are very subject to ophthalmia. For a warm climate there is nothing equal to the white or grey, broad-brimmed or "slouched," felt hat; nor is it particularly unsuitable for cold weather. We have lately seen a whole regiment, the Ulster Guards, with this form of head cover; and with one side looped up, and embellished with a cockade, the appearance was not unlike that of the old revolutionary or "continental" cocked hat, and the entire *coup d'œil*, even in a military point of view, was very fine. The slouched hat also protects the neck more effectually than any other form of hat from rain. The beard should be worn long, and there will be then no positive necessity for a cravat to protect the neck. If, however, a cravat must be worn, we must at least enter our protest against the high, leather, firm military stock, which has so long been regarded as essential to the completion of a soldier's costume.

The outer waistcoat, or vest, ought to be light and free. For this purpose, plain or twilled grey, or brown flannel, answers the purpose exceedingly well.

The coat needs to be made of a firmer material; yet while it is compact, it ought not to be heavy. Substantial, light blue broadcloth, or, in warm weather, the light, navy flannel, may serve as proper examples of the kind of material which is most suitable for an undercoat. In order to protect the front of the chest well in cold weather, it should be double-breasted. Lining the front with thick layers of cotton batting, crowding the arms into tight sleeves, and making the whole fit smoothly and snugly at the expense of the lungs, may add to the appearance of a soldier upon parade, but they are measures of doubtful utility upon a march, or in the heat of action.

The overcoat should be especially the study of the military surgeon. This is not to be worn constantly, but it is intended as a protection against the cold, the rain, and chilling damps of the night air. If properly constructed, it may also serve in an emergency instead of a blanket.

The military cloak, after the pattern of the Portugal cloak, long enough to protect the knees, made of compact duffel, firm and impenetrable to water, may serve as a sample of what might be found most useful. The United States naval military overcoat has nearly all the qualities required in this article of a soldier's dress. It is seamless, compact, firm, almost impenetrable to water, and remarkably light.

In addition to the movable cape, a capote, or hood, to be drawn over the head in a storm, and to serve as a night-cap in a bivouac, will often prove a source of comfort. According to Dr. Dumbrech, "every Turkish soldier carries this about with him; it is of strong woollen cloth; two broad straps, a yard long each, are attached to it; these, when the hood is pulled on, are brought round the jaws, covering the mouth, and forming an excellent protection against inclement weather and malaria." We have seen some lately which are made to fit snugly to the cap, and to fasten upon the visor; but they are better where open and loose, and when so constructed that they can be worn with any form of head cover.

The pantaloons in the summer may be linen or cotton, but in the winter, or in rainy seasons, woollen. They should be large and free, especially about the knees, so as in no measure to impede progression. If made somewhat smaller at the bottom, they can be easily tucked into half boots, and thus the ankles may be secured against the wet.

The question whether soldiers, at least in warm climates, ought to wear flannel or cotton next to the skin, as an under-waistcoat, has been much discussed by many medical writers, and the conclusion to which they have generally arrived has been, that flannel is preferable. It is claimed for flannel that, while, if made of some thin material, it does not add much to the actual warmth of the body, being a bad conductor of heat, it protects the surface against the influence of sudden changes of temperature, it absorbs the perspiration, and by some it is regarded as a protection of considerable value against malarial poisons, especially when worn at night. Broad flannel bands, placed around the abdomen, make tolerable substitutes for shirts.

In the winter season we regard a thick flannel under-shirt as indispensable.

Drawers may be necessary in the winter, but they are not needed in the summer.

Upon the proper construction and quality of the boots or shoes, it will be readily understood, depends much of the comfort of the soldier. The necessary elements are good leather—an article rarely to be found now-a-days—sufficient height not to chafe the ankles—a half boot is the best, with a thick and broad sole.

The socks may be cotton or woollen, but in either case it is well to place, when a long march is to be made, a piece of canton flannel between the sock and the sole of the shoe, which will serve the triple purpose of protecting the foot from the leather, of absorbing the moisture, and, by its gentle sliding motion, of preventing friction.

In addition to the points mentioned as necessary to be considered in the construction of a soldier's dress, and which relate chiefly to hygiene, there are other points in which it is to be studied, having reference solely to his immediate protection and serviceability upon the field. Any uniform which is so complicated with trappings that it cannot be easily put on in case of a surprise is objectionable, since, in the haste and confusion of the moment the soldier might omit some portion of which he stands in the greatest need. The simplest costume is, therefore, other things being equal, always the best. Garibaldi's heroes, and, during the Mexican campaign, many of our own soldiers, fought in flannel shirts and trowsers. Also all bright colors, which do not blend easily with the colors of the ground, are ill-adapted to military purposes. In this respect red and black are especially objectionable, since they form conspicuous targets for the enemy's rifles. Dark green is also visible at a great distance, and is fitted only for the costume of soldiers employed as wood rangers in Indian warfare. Even dark blue makes a clearly defined spot upon the back-ground of an ordinary landscape, and when snow covers the ground, no color is so distinctly visible. Grey, light blue, brown, or yellow, are the colors which are soonest lost in an ordinary perspective.

SECTION IV.—EXERCISE. One who is not familiar with the habits of soldiers might think it superfluous to enjoin upon them the necessity of exercise; but during a time of peace, or whenever the men are in permanent encampments, in barracks, or in cantonment, there is found to be a constant disposition to indolence; and for this reason, if we would keep them in health, and in condition for service, regular and systematic exercise is necessary.

"The Roman soldiers were exercised daily in the Campus Martius when it was fair weather, and under cover when it rained or snowed." By which they were always in complete training for active service. How much this systematic exercise is worth, every experienced officer well understands. The men ought to be summoned early in the morning, and be subjected to a severe drill, and once more, or oftener, during the day the drill should be repeated. The exercise consisting in the use of their weapons, in running, jumping, leaping, climbing, and, if possible, also in swimming. In short, the troops should be daily practised in all those exercises which might in any case prove useful in a time of war.

As far as practicable, the same exercises should be continued when soldiers are being conveyed from one post to another upon transports.

CHAPTER IV.

BIVOUAC, ACCOMMODATION OF TROOPS IN TENTS, BARRACKS, BILLETS, HUTS, ETC.

SECTION I.—BIVOUAC. A "bivouac" is the watch or guard of troops upon a field without shelter, and is only resorted to in an emergency, when the tents are not brought up, or the immediate presence of an enemy renders it unsafe to repose under their cover, as upon the eve of battle, or after a battle, when the army occupies for the night the field of the day's conquest. Sometimes also soldiers are compelled to bivouac in hurried retreats.

Little opportunity is therefore left for the selection of ground with a view to its healthfulness; yet a prudent officer will never omit to choose the most healthy as well as protected points, whenever this is consistent with the strictly military exigencies of the case. Except under an urgent necessity, he will not oblige his soldiers to bivouac upon a wet or marshy soil, where even a single night's exposure might give rise to dangerous fevers; nor when the ground is covered with snow, or the winds are cold, will the bivouac be made upon bleak and greatly exposed situations.

Possibly a position may be found, in the summer, which is dry, or in the winter, which is under the protection of a forest or of a hill, and which is at the same time convenient to water, wood, and straw or hay.

In the winter, also, unless it is important not to notify the enemy of the position of the army, where the necessary fuel can be obtained, fires may be built, and the men should be directed to lie about in groups, so as to keep each other warm, with their feet directed towards the fires. A group may be composed of three or four men, with their blankets spread out underneath and over them, resting upon their knapsacks, with their hoods drawn over their heads and ears.

Millingen suggests that when it is desirable not to show an extensive front, the fires should be "lighted in circular clusters, that the men may lie between them, and the heat be more generally diffused."

The snow, when it is of sufficient depth, may be thrown into banks or ridges, under the lee of which the men may repose; or they may lie partly imbedded in it; or they may even, where there are heavy embankments, creep into holes which they have excavated, and find themselves greatly the gainers. Millingen adds, that "incredible comfort will arise from anointing the face and ears with oil before retiring to rest or going upon duty."

"In very cold weather," says Millingen, "the sentries should only be kept on an hour; and when relieved, the men should not be permitted to lie down immediately by the fires, but be kept pacing around them till the sensation of numbness is relieved."

It is scarcely necessary to say that, in all cases, the sick and wounded should have the preference in accommodations, and that to them should be assigned the barns, or houses, or such other more comfortable places of shelter as may happen to be within reach.

Section II.—Encampment in Tents. Although the selection of the material and the plan of construction of the tents are not supposed to be in any respect under the direction of the army medical boards or of the medical staff officers, except so far as relates to the hospital tents, it is nevertheless deemed proper, in this place, to say a few words upon these points, since they are so closely connected with the comfort and hygiene of the troops.

The tents usually employed in this country by the regular army are the common ridge-pole tent, and the Sibley tent.

The ridge-pole tent is constructed of strong canvas, and it may be considered, when pitched with the proper inclination, as nearly water-proof. During heavy and continued rain-storms, however, it will generally be found to drip a little within a foot or two of the bottom, so that it is hardly a protection to those who lie near the "sod-cloth" or outer margin.

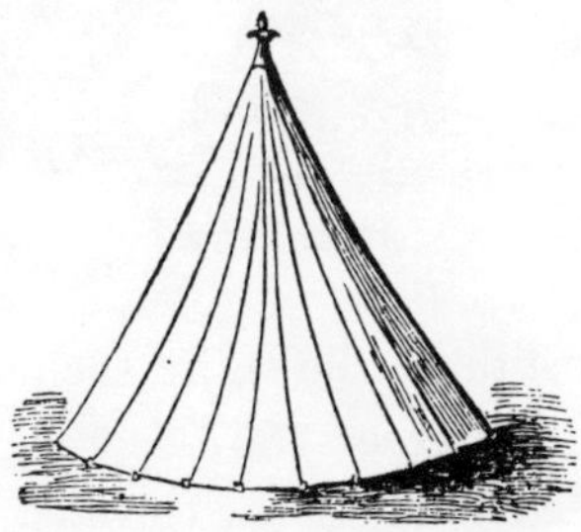

CONICAL TENT.

The following description of the Sibley tent is copied from an excellent handbook, entitled "Prairie Traveller," by Captain Marcy of the U.S.A.

"A tent has been invented by Major H. H. Sibley of the army, which is known as the 'Sibley tent.' It is somewhat similar to the Comanche lodge. But in place of the conical frame-work of poles it has one upright standard, resting upon an iron tripod in the centre. The tripod can be used to sustain cooking utensils over the fire, and, when folded up admits the wooden standard between the legs, thereby reducing the length one half, and making it more convenient for packing and travelling.

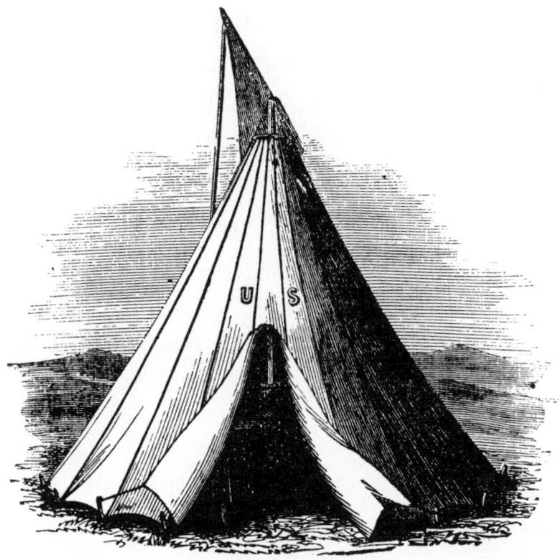

SIBLEY TENT.

"This tent constituted the entire shelter of the army in Utah during the winter of 1857–8, and, notwithstanding the severity of the climate in the elevated locality of Camp Scott, the troops were quite comfortable, and pleased with the tent.

"In permanent camps the Sibley tent may be so pitched as to give more room by erecting a tripod upon the outside with three poles, high and stout enough to admit of the tent's being suspended by ropes attached to the apex. This method dispenses with the necessity of the central upright standard.

"When the weather is very cold, the tent may be made warmer by excavating a basement about three feet deep, which also gives a wall to the tent, making it more roomy.

"The tent used in the army will shelter comfortably twelve men.

"Captain G. Rhodes, of the English army, in his recent work on Tents and Tent-Life, has given a description of most of the tents used in the different armies in Europe, but, in my judgment, none of them, in point of convenience, comfort, and economy, will compare with the Sibley tent for campaigning in cold weather. One of its most important features, that of admitting of a fire within it, and of causing a draught by the disposition of the 'wings,' is not, that I am aware, possessed by any other tent. Moreover, it is exempt from the objections that are urged against some other tents, on account of insalubrity from want of top ventilation to carry off the impure air during the night."

The "wings" spoken of by Captain Marcy are copied from the Comanche lodge, and are suspended above and to one side of the apex of the tent, for the purpose of controlling the draught of air.

As will be seen hereafter, the Sibley tent is still retained in the United States army, especially as a hospital tent; and great numbers have been recently ordered for the officers and soldiers belonging to the various volunteer regiments.

During the Crimean war, the French employed a tent which they called the "tente d'abri," and which has been highly spoken of by various writers; but it seems only suitable for the summer season, or for warm climates. "It is composed of two, four, or six square pieces of cloth, with buttons and button-holes adjusted upon the edges, and is pitched by planting two upright stakes in the ground at a distance corresponding with the length of the canvas when buttoned. The two sticks are connected by a cord passed around the top of each, drawn tight, and the ends made fast to pins driven firmly into the ground. The canvas is then laid over the rope between the sticks, spread out at an angle of about forty-five degrees, and the lower edges secured to the earth with wooden pins. This makes some defence against the weather, and was the only shelter employed by the mass of the French army in the Crimea up to October, 1855. For a permanent camp, it is usual to excavate a shallow basement under the tent, and to bank up the earth on the outside in cold weather. It is designed that upon marches the *tente d'abri* shall be taken to pieces and carried by the soldiers."

Within a few years a tent has been constructed by Mr. John Rider, of this city, 165 Broadway, composed of gutta-percha cloth, and which he has called the "tent knapsack." It resembles the "tente d'abri" of the French, and is pitched in the same manner; but while it is not so light, and perhaps not so cool in summer under a vertical sun, it possesses these two decided advantages over the French tent, namely, it is completely impervious to water, and each separate piece is easily convertible into a water-proof knapsack.

Mr. Rider's tent-knapsack was examined by the Army Medical Board assembled at Washington, and the following is an abstract from their report:—

"It is a piece of gutta-percha five feet three inches long, and three feet eight inches wide, with double edges on one side, and brass studs and buttonholes along two edges, and straps and buckles on the fourth edge; the whole weighing three pounds; two sticks, three feet eight inches long by one and a quarter inch in diameter, and a small cord. When used as a knapsack, the clothing is packed in a cotton bag, and the gutta-percha is folded round it, lapping at the ends. The clothing is thus protected by two or three thicknesses of gutta-percha, and in this respect there is a superiority over the knapsack now used by our troops.

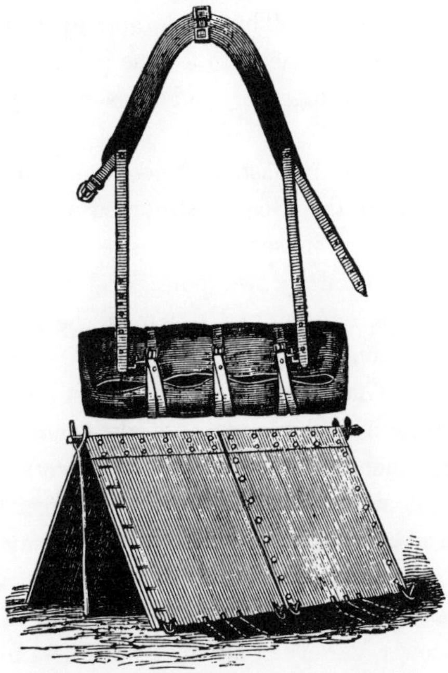

TENT-KNAPSACK. (From Prairie Trav.)

Other advantages are, that the tent-knapsack has no seams, the parts at which those in use wear out soonest; it adapts itself to the size of the contents, so that a compact and portable bundle can be made, whether the kit be entire or not; and, with the cotton bag, it forms a convenient, commodious, and durable receptacle for all a soldier's clothing and necessaries.

"On a scout a soldier usually carries only a blanket, overcoat, and, at most, a single shirt, pair of drawers, and a pair of socks, all of which can be packed in the tent-knapsack in a small bundle, perfectly protected from rain, and capable of being suspended from the shoulders and carried with comfort and ease during a march.

"2d. As a shelter. The studs and eyelets along two edges of the tent-knapsack are for the purpose of fastening a number of them together, and thus making a sheet of larger dimensions.

"A sheet formed by fastening together four knapsacks was exhibited to the Board, stretched upon a frame of wood. When used in service the sheet is to be stretched on a rope supported by two poles, or by two rifles, muskets, or carbines, and pinned down at the sides with six pins, three on each side.

"The sheet of four knapsacks is ten feet six inches long, and seven feet four inches wide, and when pitched on a rope four feet four inches above the ground, covers a horizontal space six feet six inches wide and seven feet four inches long, which will accommodate five men, and may be made to shelter seven. The sheet can also be used on the ground, and is a great protection from dampness, and as a shawl or talma; indeed, a variety of advantageous uses to which the gutta-percha sheet may be put to will suggest themselves to persons using it.

"The Board is satisfied with its merits in all the uses to which it is proposed to be put, and is of opinion that the gutta-percha tent-knapsack may be adopted in the military service with advantage."

The Army Medical Board assembled at Washington, January 19, 1860, recommended, inasmuch as the size and weight of the present *hospital* tent render it objectionable in view of its transportation, and make it difficult and oftentimes impossible to pitch it on prairies and in high winds, that in future hospital tents be made according to the pattern of the present tent, and of the same material, but smaller, and having on one end a lappel so as to admit of two or more tents being joined and thrown into one, with a continuous covering or roof. The dimensions to be these: length, fourteen feet; width, fifteen feet; height (centre), eleven feet, with a four and a half foot wall, and a "fly" of appropriate size. The ridge pole to be made in two sections after the present pattern, and to measure fourteen feet when joined. This tent is intended to accommodate from eight to ten patients. They also recommended that each regiment should be supplied with three of these hospital tents, one Sibley tent, and one common tent, all of which are designed for hospital use.

In selecting a site for the tents, the same precautious should be observed as in a bivouac, even though the tents are to remain only for a single night. But these precautions become still more important when the encampment is intended to be permanent or stationary. The position must be chosen with a view to the accessibility of water, wood, etc.; but with especial view to the comfort and healthfulness of the soldiers. In the winter the encampment may be under the shelter of a hill or of a forest; but in the summer or autumn an unbroken and somewhat elevated plane, if dry, is generally to be preferred: remote from forests, fallow fields, marshes, stagnant pools, or other well known sources of malaria. A gentle declivity, near a running stream, has the advantage of affording to the encampment the most complete drainage. If possible, let those whose duty it is to make the selection avoid an alluvial soil, or a soil composed of clay. A gravelly or rocky field is better, but no soil allows of such complete drainage as that which is sandy.

If it becomes necessary to encamp near a marsh, the tents should be closed tightly on that side which is directly exposed to the malaria.

In stationary encampments many other precautions become necessary. Permanent provisions should be made for a supply of straw or of hay, to be laid upon the ground as a protection against dampness at night. It is a common impression that it is of less consequence to protect the under side of the body than the upper; and that if the upper side is well covered, the lower, being in contact with the ground, will take care of itself. There is no more fatal error. The earth almost always contains sufficient moisture to penetrate the clothing, and even where there is no malarial poison, the dampness alone proves a frequent source of rheumatism, pleurisy, and various other inflammatory affections. A bed of straw, or of hay, or of the boughs of trees, or a wooden bunk, are almost indispensable hygienic precautions. Where it can be had, cheap and portable straw mattresses, such as are made by Mr. Rider, and which can be rolled up into a very compact form, or gutta-percha sheets and blankets, laid with the gutta-percha side down, are invaluable.

In dry weather the tents must be opened freely during the day for ventilation, and the straw or other bedding thrown out. Occasionally the straw should be replaced by that which is fresh; and if sickness is prevailing this should be done frequently.

Drains are to be dug about all of the tents. No offal is to be permitted to be thrown down before them; and no person who is well should be allowed to make a convenience of any portion of the encampment under a severe penalty.

The latrines must be placed in the rear, upon the lowest

ground; they should be narrow and deep, so as to leave as little surface for evaporation as possible; and every day a certain amount of the earth excavated in their construction should be replaced until the whole is covered in, and then new sinks should be dug. When latrines can be placed over running water this necessity is obviated.

The horses, cattle, hogs, or whatever other animals accompany the army, must be kept as remote from the encampment as possible, and no animals should be slaughtered in the immediate vicinity.

If, in spite of all these precautions, disease breaks out in the camp, the tents should be struck and the encampment changed.

SECTION III.—HUTTING. In the frontier service, in this country, where it is found impossible to procure either stone, brick, or boards for building, log huts are frequently constructed, intended to answer a temporary purpose, perhaps for a single winter, or until other building materials can be obtained. For this purpose trees of from one to two feet in diameter, being deprived of their bark, are formed into cabins or block-houses, with windows, doors, and a hole above, at one end, for the escape of the smoke and for ventilation.

The bark cannot very well be removed except during the months of June, July, or August; and if the season is unfavorable for barking, they ought to be hewn, at least upon two sides.

It is not always possible to choose the size of the timber, or the quality; but, if possible, it should be some hard or imperishable material, such as oak, cedar, red beech (the white is more perishable), pine, hemlock, ash, chestnut, or spruce: maple, poplar, basswood (linden), decay too quickly.

In no event, if it can be avoided, ought the cabin to be built of unsound timber, than which nothing can prove a more fruitful source of malaria.

To fill up the chinks between the logs, a small round stick of ash, or any other timber which cleaves easily and straight, may be split into four pieces, and laid edgewise into the spaces, where they are to be retained by wooden pegs.

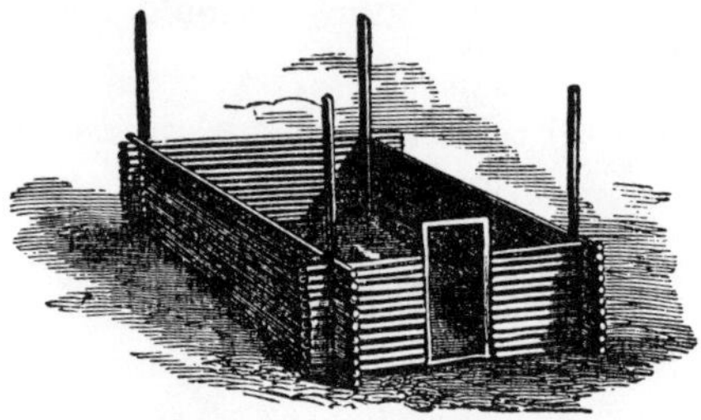

LOG HUT. (From Galton.)

A roof can be constructed of light rafters and carefully split cross-pieces of pine, and over these straw or the bark of oak, hemlock, or beech, may be laid. Shingles can be easily made of pine, hemlock, cedar, chestnut, or spruce, with the aid of a common knife.

The outside of the building may afterwards be made almost air-tight by plastering between the logs with soft clay.

The cabins should be elevated from the ground so as to allow a free ventilation underneath, whenever sufficient boards can be obtained for a floor: these open sides to be closed in on the approach of winter with logs or earth.

When the winter has fairly set in the snow may be piled up against the side of the building, and it will be found to afford an excellent protection against the driving storms and intense cold.

Where logs of sufficient size cannot be obtained, pickets

are sometimes driven into the ground, and the whole covered in after a manner similar to that first described.

Bunks are constructed of boards or twigs woven into a sort of basket, and suspended against the walls a foot or two from the floor.

If lime can be obtained, the interior should be thoroughly whitewashed.

Whether for winter or summer use, the precaution ought never to be neglected of digging a ditch entirely around each hut to catch and drain off the moisture.

Sometimes cabins are built against the side of a hill for protection, and then covered in with turf; or, as was practised in the Crimea, excavations are made in the earth, and these are simply roofed over.

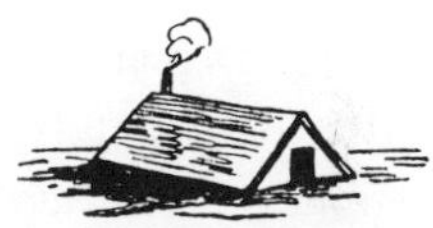

UNDERGROUND HUT. (From Galton.)

The experience of the English troops who occupied these underground tenements before Sevastopol was greatly in their favor.

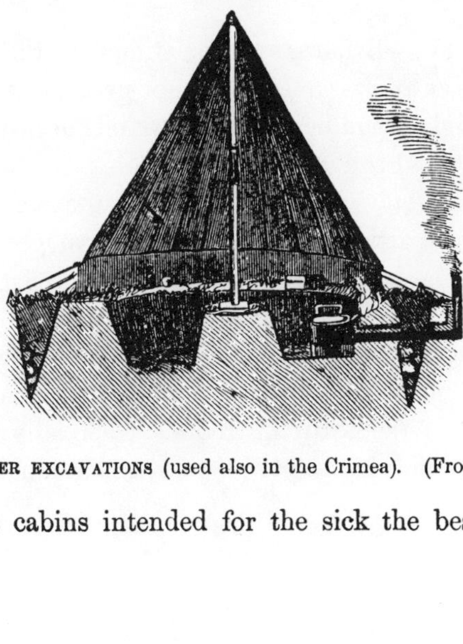

TENTS OVER EXCAVATIONS (used also in the Crimea). (From Galton.)

For the cabins intended for the sick the best situation

should be chosen. If possible, a floor should be constructed, and the same attention paid to its complete ventilation as if it were a Greenwich or a Chelsea hospital.

We have noticed, within a few days, in the "City Hall Park," a portable wooden hut, constructed by Mr. A. Derrom, of Paterson, N. J., twelve feet square, weighing 1000 pounds, but which he says may be reduced to 600 pounds. It is composed of light thin boards, laid over slight timbers, roofed with painted canvas, or gutta-percha, or India-rubber cloth, or wood, as may be preferred, and floored with boards. The whole can be taken to pieces in ten minutes and packed easily in a wagon. They may be put up separately, or any number of them can be joined together. The agent informs us that it costs $60, but we presume that they may be constructed at a much less expense if made in large numbers.

In the French and English armies board tents are now much employed, and for permanent encampments their advantages are too obvious to require to be stated.

SECTION IV.—BILLETING. Sometimes it is thought necessary, where an army is quartered in or near a town, to assign the men lodgings and board in such public or private houses as may be found convenient.

This is seldom practised except in an enemy's country, and by small parties. But the necessity ought always to be regarded as a misfortune, both to the occupant and to the soldier, especially when the billeting is prolonged. Nothing is more subversive of discipline in the army, or contributes more directly to dissipation and the consequent impairment of the health of troops. Especially is this true when the soldiers happen to be quartered at inns and drinking houses.

If billets are assigned to the men, it is the duty of the surgeon to visit and inspect them, and report the condition of the lodgings and the habits of the soldiers to the commanding officer.

SECTION V.—BARRACKS. Barracks being intended for permanent occupancy, especial care and judgment should be exercised in the selection of a site and in their construction. It is not only necessary here to regard the convenience to water and wood, the accessibility for supplies, the character of the soil in reference to drainage, the elevation, the vicinage to marshes and stagnant pools, to forests, and to fallow fields—upon all of which points information may be obtained by personal inspection—but it is proper also to ascertain by inquiry, especially from medical men in the vicinity, what diseases have been known to prevail in that locality, either constantly, annually, or at longer intervals; whether typhoid fever, intermittent fevers, the yellow fever, the cholera, or epidemic dysentery, have ever existed in that neighborhood. It is important to learn what are the prevailing winds, and whether the ground upon which the buildings are to be erected is subject to inundations, or has ever been inundated. And it might sometimes be well to ascertain whether musquitoes, or other troublesome or noxious insects, might not at certain seasons render the post uninhabitable. For this cause, old Fort Poinsett, in Florida, had to be abandoned, and Assistant-Surgeon Head reported Fort Cross as nearly untenable, in the summer months, from the same cause.

Ordinarily, unless some special objection exists, an elevated position will be preferred.

It is the duty of the medical officers not only to aid by their counsels and experience in the selection of a site for the barracks, but also in relation to their construction.

Very few, except medical men, and not even medical men unless they have paid especial attention to the subject, know much about the principles which ought to govern in the construction of a building with a view to its ventilation and healthfulness. Private dwellings, school rooms, court rooms, halls for public assemblies, prisons, asylums, barracks, and hospitals, are constantly built, often at enormous expense, with an almost total disregard to the laws of health. Indeed, it must be said, that such a disregard is the rule, and the reverse is the exception.

Barracks ought to be built of stone, brick, or iron; wood should only be employed where the building is intended for temporary occupancy, or when the more substantial materials cannot be obtained. The halls and stairways ought to be spacious, and all the ceilings lofty.

Ballingall's plan of ventilation is, to keep the halls and stairways constantly open to the outside air, by having windows at each end of the halls, extending from the ceiling to the floor, and so constructed as to be slid up or down; but never allowing the sash to come quite down to the floor. Air may be admitted also through registers in the floor of the hall from large air trunks. The air of the halls is then made to communicate with the wards by Venetian blinds over the doors, and by not allowing the doors to reach quite to the floor; also by additional holes near the floor communicating with the wards; and by holes near the ceiling on the opposite sides of the ward, which communicate directly with the external air, or with tubes which pass along under the ceiling and then enter the chimneys.

In this way, by sending the currents of air under the beds, the patients are protected from direct draughts, and the ventilation is complete. When the air enters under a bedstead it is forced off sideways so as to diffuse it more effectually.

Verandas should be constructed on each side of the building for the convenience of convalescents; and in hot climates the sick are often benefited by this exposure to a pure air. Detached from the main building should be a wash room. The sinks should also be placed remote from the barracks. The cellars for vegetables ought not to be underneath the main building.

The interior walls should be whitewashed often, and the floors scrubbed with hot water and soap, as frequently as may be necessary for the purposes of cleanliness. No doubt this practice has sometimes, especially in cold or wet seasons, been carried to an injurious extent, and especially have rheumatic patients been made to suffer from repeated exposures to a damp atmosphere.

Sometimes dry scrubbing can be properly substituted, or even a careful and thorough sweeping.

There have been erected upon the City Hall Park, in New York city, by authority of the Common Council, and under the supervision of Mr. John Corlies, architect, commodious barracks for the use of volunteer companies passing through

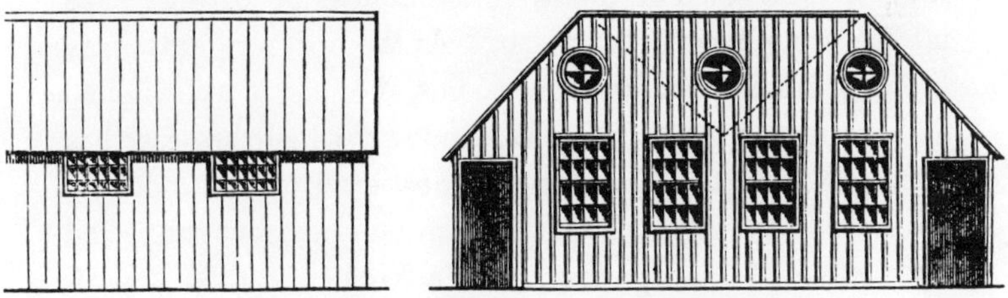

TEMPORARY BARRACKS IN CITY HALL PARK.

the city. As they have been found to answer the purpose for which they were intended in an admirable manner, a description of them may not be without its practical value.

The larger one is situated on the southwest angle of the Park, and is four hundred feet long by fifty wide, and about ten feet high at the eaves. It consists actually of two wooden frames of twenty-five feet width each, but joined so as to form a single building of fifty feet width. It contains bunks for one hundred and twenty men—the bunks being two and a half feet wide, and in four tiers. The men sleep with their feet reaching the centre of each

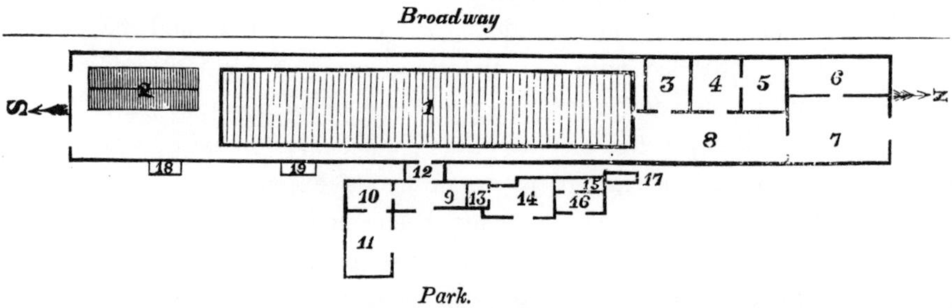

GROUND PLAN OF THE TEMPORARY BARRACKS IN CITY HALL PARK, NEW YORK.

1, Forty-one tables for eating; twenty-four seats at each table 2, One hundred and twenty bunks; four tiers; thirty in a tier. 3, 4, Store rooms. 5, 6, Officers' rooms. 7, 8, Hall. 9, Kitchen. 10, Scullery. 11, Stores and ice. 12, Passage-way. 13, 14, Rooms. 15, 16, Sutler's department. 17, Barber's shop. 18, 19, Dirty dishes.

line of bunks. There are forty tables for eating; each table seating twenty-four men. At the northern extremity are the officers' rooms, store rooms, &c. It is well lighted and ventilated by eighty-two windows, which are fixed in sliding frames, the cheapest and most expeditious mode of construction. Apart from the main building, but connected by a covered passage way, is the kitchen. This department is furnished with an excellent range, and an efficient corps of cooks, who have for some days past furnished three thousand meals per day to the volunteers. Connected with this is the room for stores and ice, and the scullery.

Adjoining the kitchen is the quartermaster's department, the sutler's department, and the barber's shop.

On the southeast angle is a smaller building, two hundred feet long by fifty wide, constructed in the same manner as the larger one. It contains bunks for seven hundred and fifty-six men, a lavatory, and latrines.

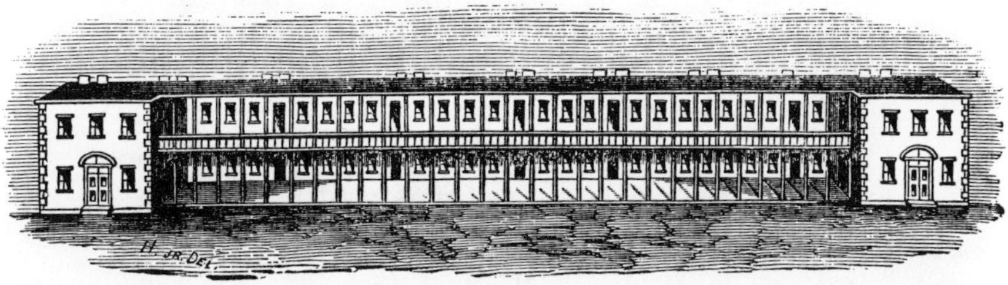

FRONT ELEVATION OF THE NAVAL BARRACKS AT BROOKLYN, N. Y.

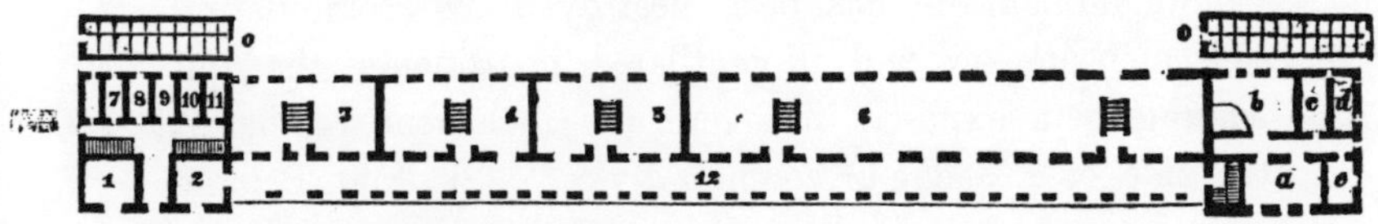

Scale 100 feet to an inch.

GROUND PLAN OF THE NAVAL BARRACKS.

1, 2, Clothes rooms. 3, 4, 5, Dormitories for eighteen men each. 6, Dining room. 7, 8, 9, 10, 11, Cells. 12, Covered walk. *a*, Laundry. *b*, Bake-house and kitchen. *c*, *d*, Store room. *e*, Pantry. *o*, *o*, Water closets and urinals.

CHAPTER V

HOSPITALS.

SECTION I.—PERMANENT HOSPITALS. In the erection of permanent hospitals, all considerations relating to location and construction must be made subordinate to the one great purpose for which they are intended, namely, the restoration of the sick to health. If it is not found possible to select a situation which is at least relatively and tolerably salubrious, it would be far better that the sick should remain without shelter, for it is undoubtedly true that "more human life has been destroyed by accumulating sick men in low and ill-ventilated apartments, than in leaving them exposed in severe and inclement weather at the side of a hedge or common dyke." Sir John Pringle used to say of large military hospitals, as constructed in his day, that they were the "graves of the army."

The chief points which are to be kept in view in the location and construction of a permanent hospital are, purity of air, ventilation, warmth in winter, coolness in summer, and durability.

Stone, brick, or iron, are preferable for their durability. In order to the complete attainment of ventilation the position should be elevated, and the form of the building should be such that all sides shall be exposed to the wind. The quadrangular form, with an interior court, is therefore the most objectionable, unless the quadrangle is composed of small detached buildings, as is the case with the great Naval Hospital at Plymouth, England If not large, it may have the form of a square, but without the interior court; or it may be constructed with a single front and without wings. But for larger establishments, a building with a single front and two short retiring wings is to be preferred. When to the main building are attached, at right angles with its extremities, retiring or salient wings, all sides are left exposed to the winds, while, at the same time, the verandas, placed along the interior, are protected measurably from the intense heats of summer and the driving storms of winter. This is the form of the fine Naval Hospital at Brooklyn, N. Y. The stellate form is equally advantageous.

If the hospital must be erected in low or damp situations, the foundations should be sunk three or four feet, and the excavation filled up with dry sand and charcoal. The basement should be high.

The same rules which have been mentioned when speaking of barracks, in relation to the construction of the halls, general ventilation, location of wash rooms, cellars, and sinks, have even a more pertinent application to permanent hospitals. The main halls, broad and lofty, ought always to traverse the building, as nearly as possible, in a straight line, from end to end. The sinks should be removed from the building, but connected by a corridor, so constructed that it may be inclosed in the winter, and left open in the summer. At least two or three doors should intersect the hall leading to the sinks, to prevent its becoming a chimney for the conveyance of the foul air to the building. Only a few water-closets should be placed within the main building. There should be a dead-house sufficiently remote, and not conspicuously located. In barracks which are not intended for invalids, and when, as is usually the case, the soldiers are a great portion of the time out of doors, it is sufficient to allow in the wards five hundred cubic feet to each man; but in hospitals more space is required. The space allowed in English hospitals averages about nine hundred and fifty feet. Hennen says eight hundred feet will do, but Ballingall thinks that if there are many bed-ridden patients they ought to be allowed one thousand feet each.

In relation to the size of the rooms, their general construction, ventilation, &c., we refer the reader to the following section, which treats of regimental or temporary hospitals, the same general rules being applicable to both.

SECTION II.—REGIMENTAL HOSPITALS. Regimental hospitals possess certain advantages over general hospitals. They are smaller, and therefore less exposed to hospital epidemics, and the patients are more immediately under the eye of the commanding officers and surgeons. The following judicious remarks of Dr. Mann, U. S. Army Surgeon, in the war of 1812, comprise nearly all that needs to be said upon this subject:

"The sick and wounded of an army, when suffered to continue with their corps, impede military operations. It has, on this account, been found expedient, in modern wars, to select some convenient post for the establishment of hospitals. Positions not too remote from the scenes of action, nor where they may be exposed to depredations of an enemy, should be chosen. A cultivated country, where milk can be procured, as well as vegetables, is preferable to towns or thick settled villages. The situation of hospitals should be at such points which least interfere with extensive military movements of an enemy and his opposing army. Although, agreeably to modern warfare, hospitals are respected by an enemy, yet, established within the compass of active movements of armies, they are exposed to be deprived of such necessary supplies as are furnished by the circumjacent countries.

"Elevated lands, which command a free circulation of air, and an abundance of good water, are preferable to plains, for the site of hospitals. They should be erected at a distance from extensive woods, where it is possible; in an open country, remote from marshes or swampy lands; and beyond the influence of winds whose currents of air are infected with miasmata generated on sunken lands, and are known to convey with them the seeds of disease.

"A military hospital which is considered temporary, built of rough materials, should never be more than one story in height.

"The attendants of a second-story house have an additional duty to perform; the sick in the wards beneath are incommoded by the necessary noise of walking on the floors over their heads. In the upper wards the observance of cleanliness is with difficulty enforced. Attendants, rather than give themselves the labor of descending a flight of stairs to execute their duty, take liberties by throwing filth from windows above, to the annoyance of patients below, without the possibility of detection.

"The wards of a military hospital should have an east and west aspect, with windows on each side. On the west, a closed passage should extend the length of the hospital, twelve feet wide, into which the doors of the several wards open. The passage should be furnished with windows, which correspond with those of the wards. This passage will be commodious for the patients able to walk, where they will be secure from cold and wet. In front of this should be an open piazza, projecting ten feet, where the patients may walk unexposed to the rays of the sun in hot weather. By means of two walls and the roof of a piazza, heat will be excluded from the rooms, which is at its highest in hot seasons after the sun has passed the meridian. These walls will also secure the wards from cold, during the severe frosts of winter.

"Wards of an extensive hospital should be thirty feet by twenty-four in dimension, and not less than eleven feet in height; which may accommodate twenty patients, if not sick with contagious diseases. This number in a ward only requires two nurses, when their diet is prepared in the kitchens. The wards of Burlington hospital (which had the reputation of being under the best regulations of any in the northern district), are twenty-four feet by twenty, and nine feet high. These rooms were found by experience to be too low. The windows of the wards should be constructed so that the upper sash may fall, and the under rise at pleasure; that when ventilating them, the air may have free access to the rooms, without passing in currents immediately over the beds of the sick.

"Convenient rooms should be appropriated for offices. One to contain hospital stores under the charge of the steward of the hospital; one for the use of the ward master, under whose care is placed the furniture and bedding; one to be improved as a dispensary; one room for a kitchen, and one for washing.

"The hospital department should be furnished with spare clothing, as well as bedding, for men who are frequently admitted destitute. During the war it was frequent that the wounded lost their clothing. Many, after the action at Little York, were received without an article except what they had on their backs, who, in consequence, were not only dirty, but covered with tribes of lice. As soon as their circumstances were reported, the commander-in-chief ordered cloth for shirts, but they could not be furnished before the men suffered for want of a change of garments.

"Each patient should be provided with a separate bed in a movable bunk. When the bunks are attached to the walls of a room, as has been sometimes the mode, they are not easily cleansed. The proper dimensions of a bunk are six feet eight inches in length, and two feet eight inches in breadth.

"Various methods have been proposed to ventilate the wards of a hospital. A hospital having east and west aspects, with single rooms, is easily ventilated; especially where the windows are made with double sashes, which rise and fall.

"Chimneys are of themselves good ventilators; no dwelling-house should be destitute of them, even in climates where fires are unnecessary to warm them. A windsail suspended over the top of a chimney by two posts and a cross piece, and its funnel let down from the top as low as the fire-place, will throw a column of fresh air into a room, which will expel the impure air through the open doors and windows. These can be employed only during the warm seasons." * * * * * * * * * * * * * *

"The following regulations were adopted in the General Hospital at Burlington, Vermont, where in no instance from its first establishment, even when the monthly reports counted from six to nine hundred men, was an infectious disease generated, or propagated.

"The washing of the floors and walls with soap and water, or lime water, was of the first importance. This was frequently repeated, especially during hot weather. In cold weather, when the wards were occupied by the sick, washing them was not only inconvenient, but hazarded the health of the patients. A coat of sand half an inch thick, or more, renewed on the floors every day, was never attended with ill consequences, but was refreshing to the sick, while it superseded the necessity of washing. Whitewashing the walls with lime and water never incommoded the sick; it sweetened the rooms and corrected infectious principles. By daily sanding the floors they were preserved not only clean but perfectly white. The opportunity of washing them was improved, when the number of sick was reduced so as to admit their removal from one ward to another. The wards were thus alternately washed and thoroughly repaired. Bunks, as soon as they were unoccupied, were removed from the wards, and after cleansing, returned. The straw of the sacks was burnt as soon as the bed was vacated. The sacks were washed once in two weeks and the straw changed. Blankets were always clean, and frequently changed. During hot seasons the windows and doors of the wards were continually open. In cold seasons the windows were opened, for a short time, repeatedly in the day; care being taken that the sick in their beds were not exposed to the direct current of air. No person was permitted to spit on the floors of the wards. Spittoons were furnished every bed, and filled with fresh sand twice a day, sometimes oftener where the patients expectorated largely. Close-stools, bed-pans, and urinals were removed as soon as employed. No culinary process was performed at the hearth of the sick wards. Attached to each ward was a closet, where the table furniture, after washing, was deposited in neat order. Each ward was furnished with a large table, constantly covered with a clean cloth of linen, the better to ensure its cleanliness, on which was placed a box with a number of little compartments, wherein were set in order the vials and medicines for the patients, each vial and parcel labelled with directions, so as to obviate mistakes.

"Attention was paid to the distribution of the sick. The wards appropriated to infectious or contagious diseases were less crowded than those occupied by patients with less important complaints. Surgical cases had rooms separated from the febrile. Venereal and itch patients were assigned to their separate wards, and not intermixed with men of different diseases.

"To guard against infection, or to obviate its generation, was of the highest importance. An infected ward was not seen where my observations were made; but it required unremitted application of those means which experience had shown to be most efficient in preventing infection—such as daily sanding the floors, ventilating the wards, and frequently washing the walls with lime and water.

"Personal cleanliness was also a means which promoted health, and obviated the generation of new diseases. At Burlington hospital, the sick, previous to admittance, were washed in tepid water in an apartment appropriated to this use; then placed in a clean bed with a clean shirt. Daily ablutions of the hands and face were ordered. The sick with febrile diseases, under the immediate direction of a surgeon, were occasionally washed or sponged with vinegar and water, at some seasons. The patients in the hospital were shaved every other day, and shirted twice in a week.

"The beds throughout the hospital were always in order whether occupied or not. If a patient left his bed ever so frequently in the day, if only for five minutes, it was immediately put in order; so that the wards were always in a condition to be visited or inspected by officers in the army.

"The inspectors generally gave a few hours' notice of their regular inspections. This was done more with a wish that the surgeons might be present at the time, than to give opportunity for preparatory arrangements. For the hospital department was not ignorant that domiciliary visits, or private inspections, were frequently made without the knowledge of the surgeons; also that confidential reports were made to government by inspectors, as a part of a system of *espionage* instituted at the war department. This was told in my hearing by an officer, when reproving one for neglect of duty. With this system we were not dissatisfied, and no officer will object to it when carried into effect without prejudice, and solely with a view to promote good discipline. But when entrusted to men who might seek their own preferment by a premeditated disgrace of others, the system was dangerous in its operation, by compelling the most efficient officers to leave the service of the army.

"The gentlemen of the hospital were not a little amused and pleasantly entertained at one time by the conduct of an assistant inspector of the line, so little acquainted with the management and arrangements of a hospital that he was ignorant of what was most fit; but willing to exhibit his talent as a critical observer, captiously censured practices designedly adopted by the director of the hospital, and recommended different methods most improper. If a department require improvement, the officers of police as well as inspection, should possess a competent knowledge of everything pertaining to it. It cannot be expected that officers of the line of an army have a correct acquaintance with all the appendages of a hospital; it seems necessary, then, that a surgeon be associated with an inspector of the line, when he executes his duty of examining the hospital department, especially when the establishment is extensive."

Iron bedsteads are to be preferred to wooden. They should not be placed quite against the wall; and about six feet square should be allowed to each bed. Curtains and valances prevent thorough ventilation, and are only depôts for dirt and contagion.

It will be well to compare with these suggestions of Dr. Mann the experience of Surgeon McLeod in the late war with Russia, and especially his observations on the use of huts as temporary hospitals. "During the early part of the war, the regimental hospital system, which I believe is peculiar to the British army, was alone followed. At a later period general hospitals were established. One large building at Balaklava, which had been a military school, was early appropriated to this purpose; and, as the number of sick increased, huts were erected to add to its accommodation. This hospital was chiefly used as a depôt for the sick about to embark for the Bosphorus, and for the treatment of sailors and native laborers. The position of the hospital was most unfortunate. In summer it was a perfect furnace; 'perched as it was in the focus of a concave mirror, of which the sides were formed of bare rock, and the bottom by the smooth water of the harbor;' and its near neighborhood to the town was a great disadvantage.

"Above Balaklava, on the face of the precipitous rocks of the coast, a number of Portsmouth and double-walled huts formed the sanitarium, to which convalescents were sent from camp. The exposed position of this hospital made it by no means an agreeable winter's residence; but in summer, its airy position, and the glorious view it commanded, afforded a most agreeable and beautiful residence for the sick who were oppressed by fever and lingering convalescence on the burning and arid plateau. This hospital contained between four hundred and five hundred beds; and the results obtained in it were unequalled, in so far as curing diseases was concerned.

"Another sanitarium was formed above the monastery of St. George, at an elevation of five hundred feet above the sea, and consisted of twelve large Chester double huts, each fitted up for twenty beds. The accommodation, both in the number of huts, and in the number of beds which each could be made to afford, could be greatly multiplied on an emergency. The construction of the huts which formed this hospital was perfect, the ventilation everything which was desirable, the water-supply sufficient, the kitchen arrangements most excellent; and, altogether, this establishment might have proved, if erected at an earlier period, one of the most useful, as it was one of the most perfect, hospitals in the East. The beautiful scenery by which it was surrounded, the cool breezes which fanned it even in the heat of summer, the agreeable walks around, and the distance it was from the turmoil of the camp, combined to render 'the monastery' as pleasing a residence as it was a favorable station for the sick.

"The general hospital in camp, which might have been termed 'the acute hospital,' as to it the men struck down in the trenches were first carried, was well situated on ground elevated between four and five hundred feet above the sea level, within the lines of the third division, and close to the extreme left of our position. It consisted at first of twenty, and latterly of thirty, Portsmouth huts. These huts were erected in four rows, facing west, leaving three broad streets between them. A space of about twelve to fifteen feet intervened between neighboring huts. This close packing was much to be regretted in the arrangement of the huts; but as they had originally been erected for the accommodation of the Fourteenth and Thirty-ninth regiments, and as space was not easily procurable where so large an army had to be encamped, the error was in a great measure unavoidable. The ground on which these huts were erected, had not been at first as carefully prepared or drained as it would have been if they had been originally erected for hospitals. Along the sides of each intervening street, deep ditches were dug, after its conversion into an hospital, to secure the drainage, and latterly the streets themselves were paved with round stones. A corps of Tartars were constantly employed in keeping the grounds clean about the huts. The cook-house and latrines were placed behind—the latter on the declivity of the hill leading down into the valley which bounded our camp from the higher plateau. These huts were erected during the winter of 1854–5, but they were not used for hospital purposes till late in the spring of the latter year. They were barely out of range, as some of the long shots from the well-known 'Crow's nest' battery came at times disagreeably near; but this propinquity favored the rapid admission of the wounded from the siege works. Each hut measured twenty-seven feet by fifteen inside, and contained, during the siege, fourteen beds; but, when the town fell, the number of beds was reduced to twelve. The air contained in these huts allowed about two hundred and sixty cubic feet to each fourteen patients. The total accommodation afforded by this hospital during the war, was four hundred and twenty beds. The arrangement of the huts was as follows:—At one end the door opened without the protection of a porch (a grave fault); at the end opposite to the door was a window; and, in some cases, there were also windows in the side walls, and a fixed one above the door. The beds were placed on either side, the heads being close to the wall, and the feet towards the centre passage, which was three feet broad; one foot and a half of open space was left between the beds. There was a stove in the centre, and ventilation traps were cut in the sides, and in many cases in the roof. The openings in the sides could be closed at night, or in stormy weather. These huts being constructed of single boards, and roofed with felt, were not impervious either to rain or cold. In wet weather, water decks had to be constructed of water-proof sheeting. Many of them were completely floored with planks; but some had merely a raised dais on either side for the beds. Peat-charcoal or lime was frequently strewn beneath the planking, and the most scrupulous cleanliness was rigidly enforced. The men's kits were stowed in huts set apart for the purpose, so as to relieve the wards as much as possible from incumbrance. The bedsteads and bedding were excellent, the provision of medical comforts good, and the cooking passable; so that on the whole, a better field hospital in the camp of an active army I suppose never existed.

"To an hospital so situated, one whose object was so temporary, and whose inmates were so liable to fluctuation, we cannot apply the same rules of criticism that we adopt when discussing the merits of more permanent establishments. That the patients were often crowded, that the proper amount of air was not measured out to each, that many of the refinements of a London hospital were wanting, may be admitted; but I doubt whether a better hospital could be provided three thousand miles from England, in a crowded camp, in a houseless region, before an active and energetic enemy, and almost in the vortex of the strife. The ventilation was much better, even at the times of greatest crowding, than could be supposed possible; and, as the wards were seldom full, except for short periods after some of the great battles, or assaults, it was generally beyond cavil. Unquestionably the beds were too close; the huts were too near one another, and erected within the precincts of a crowded camp; and, in summer, the heat was great; but while I most willingly allow that there was much in all this which was reprehensible, still I cannot conscientiously say that I had often reason to complain of the close air of the wards. The thinness of the walls of the huts, and the numerous air-traps cut in them, did much to prevent the formation of a dangerous atmosphere, but gave rise to disagreeable currents of air, of which the men often complained. This could not be effectually overcome by any lining short of wood. The absence of porches to the doors greatly favored these draughts. In winter, the huts were very cold and uncomfortable, notwithstanding the pains we took to hang up blankets and bed-covers round the beds."

SECTION III.—FIELD OR FLYING HOSPITALS are Medical Detachments which accompany the army, whether upon the march or in engagements. During an engagement the flying hospital is posted, by order of the senior Staff Surgeon, at some convenient point near the field of battle, in order that the wounded may receive early succor. Occasionally the regular hospital tent is employed as the depôt, at other times a barn, shed, or house may be chosen; but if the weather is pleasant, it may be sufficient to select a spot which is protected from the fire of the enemy, and where water and shade may be found. When tents or buildings are not resorted to, the term "flying hospital" continues to apply to the medical corps, in whatever direction it may move, or wherever it may chance to be.

At these points the wounded receive their first succor, and most of the minor dressings are made, and some of the major; after which, they are sent to the rear, to be placed in such temporary hospitals or permanent, as may be provided for them.

In the British Crimean service, during most of the time occupied in the siege, Assistant Surgeons gave the first attention to the wounded before they were sent to the rear. But at the time of an assault, Staff Surgeons were advanced to the ravines, and performed such operations as were necessary on the spot, and attended to the transmission of the wounded to the hospitals. The French also adopted much the same method. They placed ambulances in the ravines, close to the trenches, where balls were extracted, dressings made, &c., after which the wounded were passed to the divisional ambulances.

CHAPTER VI.

PREPARATIONS FOR THE FIELD.

GUTHRIE says, "A surgeon without his apparatus and equipments is little better than a battery of artillery without ammunition." Yet it is not possible that Surgeons employed in army service should be as well supplied with instruments, apparatus, and medicines as in civil practice; nor that the sick or wounded soldier should receive that attention, or enjoy those comforts of warm and abundant clothing, soft beds, and easy conveyance to which he has in many cases been accustomed; and especially is this true in relation to the immediate provisions for the sick and wounded after a battle, or upon the march. While everything ought to be provided, consistent with the means of the Government, the rapidity of movement of the troops, the peculiarities of the country, the climate, and the nature of the warfare, yet it must be seen that to some extent a soldier's privations must continue even when he becomes a patient. Many things, usually regarded as eminently desirable, must be sacrificed to the necessities of the service. What is necessary must, if possible, be supplied—but luxuries must be left behind; compactness being generally a primary consideration in everything relating to the army when in motion or in active service.

In the United States army each Regimental Surgeon is allowed for three months service—

1 Sponge-holder, for the throat (Buck's).
8 Cupping Glasses.
8 Tin Cups, for the same purpose.
6 Thumb Lancets (in cases).
1 Spring Lancet.
1 Set of Pocket Instruments.
12 Whalebone Probangs.
4 Scarificators.
1 Set of Splints (major) Welch's.
1 Stomach Pump and case.
4 Enema Syringes, of which
  1 Davidson's,
  1 Hard Rubber, 6 oz.
8 Glass Penis Syringes.
8 India-rubber Penis Syringes.
1 Set of Teeth Extracting Instruments.
1 Tongue Depressor (on a hinge).
8 Field Tourniquets.
2 Spiral Tourniquets (Petit's).
6 Hernia Trusses.

In addition to the above, each medical officer is supplied with five cases of instruments; which, so long as the officer remains in the service, are his own private property, to be returned, however, to the department whenever he leaves the army; and for the complete and serviceable condition of which he is at all times responsible.

The following is a list of the instruments with which these several cases are furnished:

AMPUTATING.

1 Capital Saw.
1 Metacarpal Saw.
1 Capital Amputating Knife.
1 Medium " "
1 Small " "
1 Large Catling.
1 Small "
1 Scalpel.
1 Tenaculum.
1 Artery Needle.
1 " Forceps.
1 Bone "
1 Spiral Tourniquet.
12 Surgeon's Needles.
1 Mahogany Case, brass bound.
1 Gutta Percha Pouch.

TREPHINING.

2 Trephines.
1 Scalpel, with Raspitor.
1 Hey's Saw.
1 Elevator.
1 Brush.
1 Mahogany Case, brass bound.

EXSECTING.

1 Bone Forceps (Liston's).
2 Bone Forceps, sharp, assorted.
1 Bone Forceps, for sequestra.
1 Chain Saw.
1 Chisel.
1 Gouge.
1 Lenticular Knife.
2 Spatulas, protecting.
1 Trephine, small crown.
1 Ecraseur.
1 Mahogany Case, brass bound.
1 Gutta Percha Pouch.

GENERAL OPERATING.

1 Metacarpal Saw.
1 Trocar.
1 Ball Forceps.
1 Gullet "
1 Artery "
1 Dressing "
2 Scissors, straight and curved.
1 Artery Needle, with 4 points.
12 Surgeon's Needles.
1 Tourniquet.

1 Small Amputating Knife.
1 " Catling.
3 Bistouries.
1 Hernia Knife.
3 Scalpels.
1 Cataract Knife.
1 " Needle.
1 Tenaculum.
1 Double Hook.
6 Steel Bougies, silvered, double curve, Nos. 1 and 2, 3 and 4, 5 and 6, 7 and 8, 9 and 10, 11 12.
6 Wax Bougies, Nos. 2, 4, 6, 8, 10.
3 Silver Catheters, Nos. 3, 6, 9.
6 Gum-elastic Catheters, Nos. 1, 3, 5, 7, 9, 11.
2 Mahogany Cases, brass bound.
1 Gutta Percha Pouch.

POCKET.

1 Large Scalpel.
1 Small "
1 Artery Forceps.
1 Bull-dog Forceps.
1 Curved "
1 Dressing "
1 Needle.
1 Sharp-pointed Bistoury.
1 Probe-pointed "
1 Long Probe-pointed Bistoury.
1 Straight Scissors.
1 Knee "
1 Flat-curved Scissors.
1 Gum lancet.
1 Tenaculum.
1 Tenotomy Knife.
1 Abscess Lancet.
1 Exploring Needle.
1 Exploring Trocar.
1 Seton Needle.
1 Spatula.
2 Probes.
1 Director.
1 Double Canula.
1 Comp'd Silver Catheter.
6 Surgeon's Needles.
1 Artery Needle.
1 Morocco Case.

For the whole of which a substantial leather trunk is provided.

About eighty different medicines are furnished as a three months' supply to each regiment, a few medical books, hospital stores, and bedding.

Most of the medicines used in the United States Army are manufactured and supplied by E. R. Squibb, M.D., late of the United States Naval Laboratory, at his laboratory, 149 Furman Street, Brooklyn. The name of Dr. Squibb is a complete guarantee of their excellence to all who have a personal acquaintance with the man, or who have used his drugs. Of one thing we may be certain, therefore, however poorly our soldiers may be clothed or fed, they are in no danger from impure or adulterated drugs.

The schedule entitled "Furniture and Dressings," is as follows:

Bandages, roller assorted	doz.	14	
" suspensory, assorted,	no.	12	
Binders' boards	no.	18	18 inches by 4.
Buckets, leather	no.	4	BANDAGES.
Corks, assorted	doz.	12	1 doz., 1 in. wide, 1 yd. long.
Corkscrews	no.	2	2 " 2 " 3 "
Cotton batting	lb.	2	2 " 2½ " 3 "
" wadding	lb.	2	1 " 3 " 4 "
Flannel (red)	yds.	5	½ " 3½ " 5 "
Hatchets	no.	2	½ " 4 " 6 "
Hones	no.	1	4 inches by 1, in wood.
Ink, 2-ounce bottles	no.	12	
Knapsack, hospital	no.		According to pattern.
Lanterns	no.	4	
Lint	lb.	8	
Litters and stretchers, hand	no.		According to pattern.
" horse	no.		
Measures, graduated, assorted	no.	4	6 oz., 2 oz., minim.
Medicine chests	no.		
" cups and glasses	no.	6	2 cups to 1 glass.
" panniers	no.		
Mess chests	no.		
Mills, coffee	no.	2	
Mortars and pestles, wedgewood,	no.	2	Small.
Muslin	yds.	20	
Needles, sewing	no.	25	Assorted, in a case.
Oiled silk or gutta percha tissue, or India rubber tissue	yds.	8	
Pans, bed	no.	2	Of hard India rubber or other material. Shovel.
Paper envelopes, assorted	no.	100	50 letter, 25 note, 25 large. "Official Business" printed on each.
Paper, wrapping	quires.	6	
" writing	quires.	12	2 foolscap, 6 letter, 4 note, white; blue ruled.
Pencils, hair	no.	24	
" lead	no.	12	Of Faber's make, No. 2.
Pens, steel	doz.	4	
Pill boxes (wood)	papers.	2	
" (tin)	no.	6	
Pins, assorted	papers.	4	Large and medium.
Razors	no.	1	
Razor strops	no.	1	
Scales and weights, apothecary's	sets.	1	
Scissors	no.	4	
Sheep skins, dressed	no.	4	
Silk, surgeon's	oz.	½	
Silk, green	yds.	1	
Spatulas	no.	6	
Sponge (washed)	lb.	1	
Tape	pieces.	4	

Thread, linen	oz.	2	
Tiles	no.	2	
Towels	no.	40	
Twine	lb.	½	
Urinals	no.	4	
Vials, assorted	doz.	4	1 oz. to 2 oz.
Wafers (½ ounce boxes) . .	no.	1	
Wax, sealing	sticks.	2	

Patent lint is used exclusively in the United States Army, but scraped, ravelled, or pulled lint will do as well; or beaten flax. The latter may be had of Tiemann & Co., Instrument Makers, New York, and it may be obtained at the moderate price of 65 cts. per lb. It is light, porous, and unirritating, and by many surgeons is preferred to lint.

The material used for bandages is plain, cheap, unbleached muslin. It ought to be rolled by a machine, in order that it may form a small and hard roller easily managed by the hand, and that it may occupy as little space as possible.. Each roller should have upon it a label indicating the length and width of the piece, and the whole should be then neatly done up in packages marked "7 doz. rollers, assorted."

The furniture of the "mess chest" mentioned in the last schedule, consists of

8 Basins, tin.
2 Boxes, pepper and salt.
6 Cups, tin.
4 Canisters (for tea, coffee, sugar, and butter).
2 Dippers and ladles.
1 Grater.
1 Gridiron.
1 Kettle, tea, iron.
12 Knives and forks.
6 Mugs (Britannia, half-pint).
1 Pan, frying.
1 Pan, sauce.
8 Plates (6) and dishes, (2) tin.
1 Pot, iron.
2 Pots, coffee and tea, tin.
12 Spoons, iron, (table [6] and tea [6]).
1 Tray, tin.
6 Tumblers, tin.

For general and post hospitals, considerable addition is made to the articles enumerated, and the supply is much larger, being estimated usually for one year.

We have recently had constructed a "Field Case," designed to be used by the surgeons especially when upon the field of battle. Our object has been to comprise within a single case all the instruments which are likely to be needed in an emergency, and which case may be sufficiently compact and light to be easily carried from one point to another. It is not intended to supply all the wants of a hospital, or to complete the armamentarium of the regimental surgeon, but only to obviate the necessity of carrying several cases where only a few instruments are needed.

Messrs. Wade & Ford, Instrument Makers, 85 Fulton street, and also Geo. Tiemann & Co., 63 Chatham street, New York, have put them up very neatly, and made for them a leather case, after the pattern of those used in the army. These instruments are provided mostly for amputation, trephining, ligature of arteries, and simple dressings; since these constitute the major part of the operations usually made upon the field, unless we except the temporary dressing of fractures.

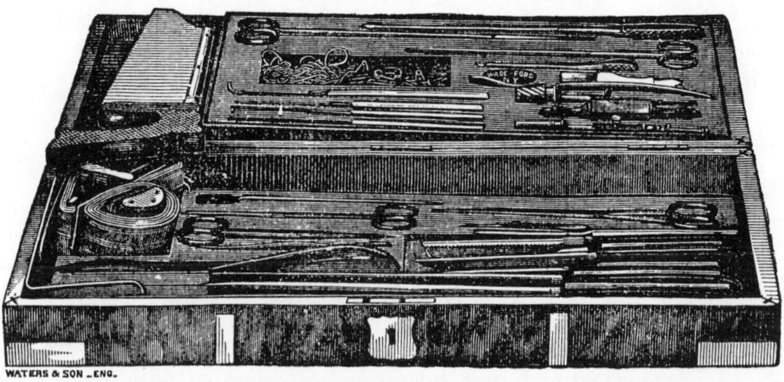

THE AUTHOR'S FIELD CASE.

The following is a schedule of the instruments furnished to the medical officers of the United States Navy:

AMPUTATING SET.

1 Long Knife.
1 Short "
1 Catling.
1 Metacarpal Saw.
1 Scalpel.
1 Tenaculum.
1 Saw.
1 Bone Forceps.
1 Artery "
6 Needles.
1 Tourniquet.

TREPHINING CASE.

2 Trephines.
1 " Brush.
1 Hey's Saw.
1 Elevator.
1 Set Urethral Dilators, plated (6 instruments), graduated at both ends.
2 Silver Catheters.
1 Stomach Pump, and Self-injecting Apparatus.

MINOR OPERATING CASE.

4 Scalpels.
1 Sharp Bistoury.
1 Blunt-pointed "
1 Hernia "
1 Aneurism Needle.
1 Tenaculum.
1 Artery Forceps.
1 Pair Scissors.
6 Small Needles.
1 Bullet Forceps.
1 Curved Trocar.
1 Straight "
1 Plated Syringe, with fittings for Hydrocele and the Ear.
1 Hone.
1 Probe.
1 Instrument Case.
1 Gutta Percha Cover.

The minor splints recommended for the army are coarse, rather thick, unglazed binder's board, cut into pieces of eighteen inches by four, for the convenience of packing, and splints made of calfskin, veneered with white wood, the latter being subsequently split into strips of about half an inch in width, so as to combine a certain degree of flexibility with the requisite firmness. The "major" splints are a complete set of Welch's splints, made mostly of gutta-percha veneered with some light and slightly flexible wood. There is also furnished one sheet of gutta-percha (see Schedule) for occasional use as splints.

The splints furnished for the navy are

1 double inclined plane.

1 long splint, for fractures of the lower extremities, with a belt and perineal pad and strap.

1 short, curved splint, for the inside of the thigh.

2 curved splints, for general use.

All of which have pads fitted and tied on them.

1 set of leathered wooden splints (same as in the army).

2 sheets of cotton wadding, and a package of tow accompanying each set of splints. The whole inclosed in a substantial box.

"The double inclined plane has the lower part so arranged as to be easily detached and used separately as a fracture box when required.

"It is also provided with large buttons on the bottom, which when turned cross-wise make the apparatus sit more firmly on the mattress.

"The long splint for the lower extremities is adapted for the use of an adhesive plaster extending band. A strip of adhesive plaster, about two inches wide, is to be applied to the limb, in the direction of its axis, from near the seat of fracture, down one side and up the other, leaving a loop or stirrup under the sole of the foot. The whole is then enveloped with a roller bandage, applied with a moderate degree of firmness. A thin piece of board, about two inches square, is made to adhere to the inside of the loop or stirrup, at the sole of the foot; and around this, and over the hook of the splint, a piece of tape is passed, by which to make extension.

"A pocket is made in the belt, to receive the upper end of the splint; and the buckles on the outside of the pocket receive the ends of the perineal straps for counter-extension.

"To adapt the splint to opposite sides, it is only necessary to take out the hook and adjust it so that the opening looks upward."

These splints, contrived and arranged by Drs. Bache and Squibb, of the navy, constitute the most compact and serviceable set which we have ever seen, and might very well be adopted as a model for either military, naval, or private practice.

For such regiments as cannot conveniently furnish themselves with all the splints recommended by the Army and Navy Medical Boards, we would advise the binder's board, eighteen pieces (see Schedule)—two nests of splints made of undressed sole leather, one nest of plain wooden splints (white wood, pine, or ash), and one sheet of gutta-percha.

A "nest" of splints may be prepared as follows: The first and largest splint, eighteen inches by four; the second, sixteen by three and a half; the third, fourteen by three; the fourth, twelve by two and a half; and the fifth, ten by two. Reducing the splints each time by two inches in length, and half an inch in breadth.

As an adhesive plaster, the surgeon will need, when upon the field, either Tallman's or Husband's isinglass plaster, neither of which requires the aid of heat in its application, but only needs to be moistened slightly upon one surface.

The Army Medical Board, convened at Washington, November, 1859, recommended the adoption of a hospital knapsack, to be carried by a hospital orderly upon the march or in battle, who is habitually to follow the medical officer. The knapsack to be made of light wood; divided into four compartments or drawers, and covered with canvas after Colonel Buchanan's model knapsack. The purpose of this is to carry, in an accessible shape, such instruments, dressings, and medicines, as may be needed in an emergency on the march or in the field. The dimensions of the hospital knapsack to be those of the ordinary knapsack. These are regularly furnished for each regiment; but they are now made of willow.

CONTENTS OF HOSPITAL KNAPSACK.

1 quart Castor Oil.	1 oz. Zinci Sulph. (Squibb's.)
1 lb. Cerati Simplicis.	¼ oz. Argenti Nitr. fused. "
4 oz. Chloroform. (Squibb's.)	2 oz. Alum. (Squibb's.)
4 oz. Ext. Ipecac. Fld.	2 yds. Emp. Ichthyocollæ (with Meds. 17 lb).
4 doz. Pills Cathartic Co.	2 yds. Emp. Adhesivi.
2 " " Mass. Hydr. 5 gr.	½ lb. Lint.
2 " " Opii.	2 pieces Sponge.
4 " " " gr. i. and Camphor gr. ii.	4 doz. Bandages, assd.
4 " " Quiniæ Sul. gr. iij.	2 yds. Flannel.
1 oz. Potass. Iodidi.	4 Binder's Boards (4 × 18 inches) doubled.
½ oz. Quiniæ Sulph.	1 Field Tourniquet.
4 oz. Spts. Ether Comp. (Squibb's.)	2 Lead Pencils.
4 oz. " Terebinth.	1 qr. Note Paper.
4 oz. Tinct. Opii.	1 paper Pins and 1 ps. Tape.
4 oz. " " Camph.	

The knapsack weighs, when empty, six pounds, and when supplied with the articles above enumerated, its weight, including the bottles, is about eighteen pounds.

The following excellent suggestions, taken from a contemporary daily journal, deserve to be remembered:—

"In the course of a battle, the gunners, and in fact all engaged, are subjected to injuries of the ear, by the heavy and long sustained discharge of powerful artillery. Numerous cases of ruptured membrane, with more or less permanent deafness, will be found among the returning soldiers. In the artillery, the effect of position with reference to the gun is peculiar. Those men who stand nearest the muzzle *feel* the report most, but all who are to the leeward suffer more than those to the windward. Let the Medical Staff of each regiment keep prepared a quantity of glycerine, mixed with belladonna, say in about the proportion of forty grains of the latter to the ounce of glycerine oil. Let each gunner be provided before an engagement with wool or cotton (the former is preferable), saturated with the mixture, to place in his ears. It will not prevent his hearing the word of command, or the drum, and will prevent a great deal of injury. The therapeutic of the preventive, medical men will perceive, as it forms a coating over the membrane, which can be easily cleansed by a little warm water, and will effectually prevent the vibration of the air striking injuriously upon it. It would also be useful to those exposed to dampness, when camping out at night, the organ in question being extremely sensitive to the night air. By taking this precaution the deafness to which gunners are now so liable may be prevented."

CHAPTER VII.

HYGIENIC MANAGEMENT OF TROOPS UPON THE MARCH.

FIFTEEN miles per day is considered a fair average for infantry; and upon long marches, ten miles, including all the necessary delays, is accounted good travelling. This will depend much, however, upon the nature of the country, the season of the year, as well as upon whether the troops are newly recruited, or old soldiers accustomed to hardships and to travel.

Some of the longest marches of infantry upon record have been made by American troops. During the first year of the Mexican war, Gen. Kearney was placed in command of the "Army of the West," with instructions to conquer New Mexico and California. He left Fort Leavenworth, Kansas, in June, and after a journey of nine hundred miles over the great plains and mountain ranges, arrived at Santa Fé, the capital of New Mexico, on the 18th of August. In the year 1860, a large portion of the Seventh Regiment marched from Camp Floyd, U. T., to Fort Buchanan, New Mexico, having travelled one thousand miles, and spent one hundred and forty days on the road. But the most unprecedented march of infantry was made by the gallant old Sixth, in 1859, which left Fort Leavenworth, Kansas, for California, a distance of two thousand eight hundred miles, and was one hundred and ninety days on the road, of which one hundred and sixty-two were actually passed in marching, being at the rate of about eleven miles per day.

Even in warm climates, it is better that the sleep of the soldier should not be broken before day, as what is gained by the avoidance of the heat of the midday is more than lost by the interruption of the natural rest. A light breakfast of coffee and bread, or potatoes, ought always to precede the march. The first hour the troops should not march more than three miles; and after an interval of fifteen minutes, during which they should be encouraged to throw off their knapsacks and recline, they be again set in motion. The distance may be increased the second hour to about three and a half miles; and after resting again the line of march may be resumed at the rate of four miles per hour. This ought never to be exceeded, except in forced marches. After three hours' march, if in summer, the troops should be allowed to rest until the heat of the sun is less oppressive, the travel to be commenced again in the afternoon.

During the midday rest, and while dinner is preparing, each soldier would do well to take off his shoes and socks, and wash his feet, if water is accessible, so as to remove the acrid perspiration and dirt. He ought especially to wash between the toes, and by this means he will do much towards the prevention of excoriations and soft corns. It is sometimes advantageous to change the socks from one foot to the other, so that their seams or folds shall press upon new points. When the heels become tender, or ulceration is threatened, they should be protected with common adhesive plaster.

It is unnecessary to say that the soldier's clothing ought to be suited to the climate and season, and that he should carry as little weight about his person as possible. The English troops carry on an average, including knapsack, haversack, and firelock, between fifty and sixty pounds;

but in the American army, this is reduced to about forty pounds. If this amount can be diminished in any way consistent with the necessities of the case it would be better. The knapsack ought never to weigh over seventeen pounds; and it is worthy of remark, that with one extra shirt, and one extra pair of socks, the soldier's wardrobe is more generally found clean than when he is supplied with a greater number of changes. If he has but one extra shirt he loses no opportunity to make it clean, if he has two he neglects to avail himself of the best chances for washing and drying.

The knapsack should be "slung," and not strapped tightly to the back, for it is better that it should "roll" a little, than that it should restrict the free motions of the arms. The breast-strap should never be buckled, except when the shoulder-straps begin to gall the arm-pits; it always impedes somewhat the action of the muscles of respiration, and in long or rapid marches it becomes a serious inconvenience. The chest should, as far as possible, be left free for expansion, but the muscles of the loins are supported and invigorated by being well girt about with a broad and firm band.

Indians walk with their toes directly in front of the heel, and experience shows that a man walks faster and longer with his feet in this position than with the toes turned out. The "toeing in," as it is called, enables the person to avail himself most completely of the action of the muscles of the leg and foot. Unencumbered with weight, a man walks easier with his trunk erect, and set square over his haunches; but with a knapsack and gun, it is better to incline a little forwards, especially in rapid progression.

The length of the military step in the British line, is

thirty inches, but this is suited only to men of full stature, say five feet eight inches, or six feet; nor is it suited to marching *en route*. In the American service the rule is twenty-eight inches for common, and thirty-three for quick time. From twenty-three to twenty-six inches will be found the most convenient for most men in the "route step."

To avoid excessive thirst, a full draught of cold water should be taken before starting, and then the mouth should be kept closed during the march as much as possible. The Arabs keep their mouths covered with a cloth. Holding a smooth pebble in the mouth, or chewing a green leaf, will alleviate the thirst somewhat. Simply moistening the mouth occasionally with water is better than drinking often or freely.

If the water is muddy it may be filtered through a sponge, or a cloth of any kind; or by rolling a handful of grass in the form of a cone, and having dipped it into the pool, allowing it to drip from one end. When a greater supply is needed, it may be obtained in the following manner: a number of holes may be bored in a cask, and having removed the bottom from another and smaller cask, it is to be placed inside the first; fill in the space between the two with grass, hay, straw, moss, tow, wool, sponge, charcoal, sand, or pebbles, and then sink it into the water. A stout canvas bag, kept open by a hoop, and sunk by the weight of a stone, will answer tolerably well. If the water is simply turbid, alum will settle it very quickly, leaving no taste of alum in the water: a teaspoonful is sufficient to render clear a pailful of turbid water. Galton says this plan is adopted very generally in India. A piece of alum merely moved about in a vessel of water will accomplish the same purpose.

Putrid water, filled with vegetable matter and animalcula, ought to be boiled, with a little charcoal in the vessel, before drinking, if possible. "The Indians," says Galton, "plunge hot iron into putrid and muddy water." As the scum rises to the surface it should be removed.

Water can be kept tolerably cool by inclosing the can or bottle in which it is carried in a wet cloth, and allowing it to evaporate. Leather being slightly porous, and allowing a little of the water to evaporate slowly from its surface, keeps the contents more cool than gutta-percha, india-rubber, or metal.

A few drops of vinegar, or of lemon juice, added to the water, to give it a relish, is better than brandy, and it is much more likely to allay thirst; yet, if used too freely, it may occasion a colic or a diarrhœa.

The amount of the rations should be considerably increased when men are upon a march, or in active duty; and they ought to have at least three meals per day, two of which should be substantial, and composed in a great measure of meat. Christison has shown that a man in sedentary life requires only about seventeen ounces per day of real nutriment, but that when actively employed, in rough work, he demands from twenty-eight to thirty ounces, or even more. Of course the most compact and nutritious aliments are those which should be selected.

We do not think it safe ever to trust soldiers with opium, morphine, or medicines of any kind, since there are more chances that they will use them injudiciously, than at proper times or in proper quantities.

For many other matters relating to the comfort and health of the soldier upon the march, we will refer the reader to the chapter on Hygiene.

CHAPTER VIII.

CONVEYANCE OF SICK AND WOUNDED SOLDIERS.

For the purpose of conveying wounded soldiers from the field of battle to the several depots where the regimental hospital corps are assembled, as well as for the purpose of transporting them upon marches, or from one depot or hospital to another, three principal kinds of conveyances have been employed. *First*, those which may be handled by men, called "hand-bearers," "litters, or sedans;" *second*, mules or horses with panniers; and *third*, wheel carriages, which require the aid of horses, mules, or bullocks.

Section I.—"Hand-litters." Gen. Jackson recommended and adopted occasionally, a very simple method of conveying the sick, in his expeditions against the Indians, viz. to suspend a bull's hide between two muskets, upon which the patient was carried by two or four men, as the case might require. Soldiers' blankets might serve the same purpose, in case of necessity, especially if they were made with strong loops upon the opposite margins; in which case they might be doubled upon themselves so that all the loops should be upon the same margin. Through these loops a gun might then be thrust, and another gun through the doubling.

Dr. George Suckley, late Surgeon in the United States Army, says, that he has occasionally, in frontier service, constructed a temporary stretcher of two poles cut from the forest; these being laid upon the edges of a blanket, rolled in, and finally made fast with strong twine, by puncturing the blanket at intervals of a foot along the sides of the poles and tying the twine strongly on the outside.

A very simple and ingenious method of conveyance is to make use of the soldier's overcoat as a sacking. The sleeves being turned inside out, and a musket thrust through each sleeve, the wounded man is laid upon the coat and it is then buttoned together in front. Two men standing between the ends of the guns may now lift him easily; but the conveyance will be made more secure by detaching the leather slings from the guns and passing them under the body, or if they are unnecessary here, they may be employed to cross over the shoulders of the carriers. Canvas may be substituted for the overcoat, guns being used for poles, as we learn from Retzius, is the practice sometimes in the Swedish army.

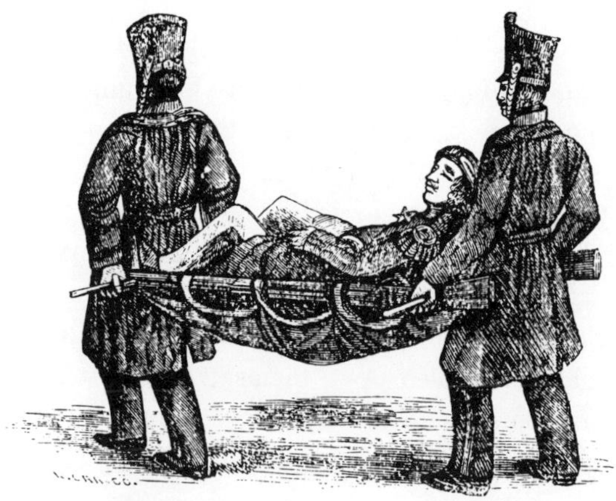

HAND-LITTER, MADE WITH GUNS. (From Galton.)

To all of these methods there exists the serious objection that they have no "traverses" or "stretchers" to prevent the bottom from sinking down, while at the same time the guns or poles are pressed uncomfortably against the hips of the bearers.

Ballingall thinks that Dr. Millingen has suggested the "most simple, efficient, and practicable" contrivance for the conveyance of the wounded which has yet been devised. It consists of two parallel poles, separated by two traverses or stretchers, with short legs, and supporting a canvass bottom. The poles of these bearers, when not employed for this purpose, and armed with pikeheads, form weapons of offence and defence to the men of the hospital corps when escorting wounded or guarding hospital stores or provisions. Each individual of this corps should be armed with one of these pikes, furnished with one of the traverses strapped upon his knapsack, and one of the canvas bottoms girted round his waist; and any two of them meeting together, will be enabled in a few minutes to equip a light and efficient bearer, capable of carrying off a wounded man with all the comfort of which his situation admits: his pack being placed under his head as a pillow, and his firelock slung from the side of the bearer by means of loops attached to it for this purpose. Dr. Millingen also proposes that each transporter should be furnished with sling-belts, by which the bearer will be slung from the shoulders and more easily carried.

The hand-litters employed in the United States Army are

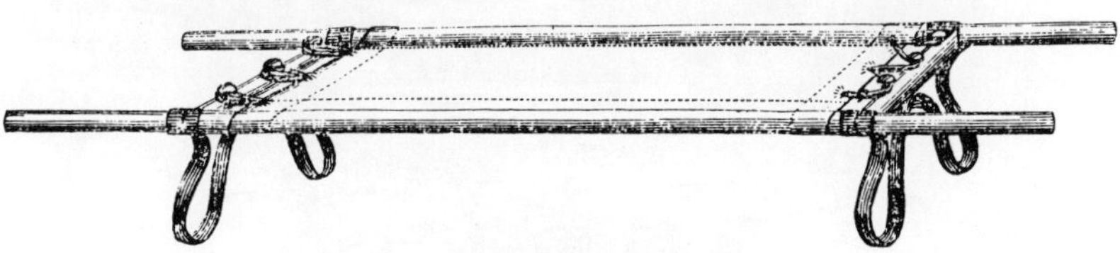

UNITED STATES ARMY HAND-LITTER.

composed of two light but strong poles made of ash, each eight feet ten inches long, and one inch and three quarters in diameter, with cross-pieces six feet apart and twenty-nine inches in length, to keep the poles from falling together; across this frame is stretched a firm canvas, made fast at either end by loops hitched to pins on the cross-pieces. The whole can be easily separated and rolled into a compact form for transportation.

Says Galton in his "Art of Travel:" "If a man be wounded or sick, and has to be carried along upon the shoulders of others, make a stretcher for him in the Indian fashion; that is to say, cut two stout poles, each eight feet long, to make its two sides, and three other cross-bars of two-and-a-half feet each to be lashed to them. Then supporting this ladder-shaped frame-work *over* the sick man as he lies in his blanket, knot the blanket up well to it; and so carry him off, palanquin-fashion. One cross-bar will be just behind his head, another in front of his feet; the middle one will cross his stomach, and keep him from falling out; and there will remain two stout handles for the carriers to lay hold of.

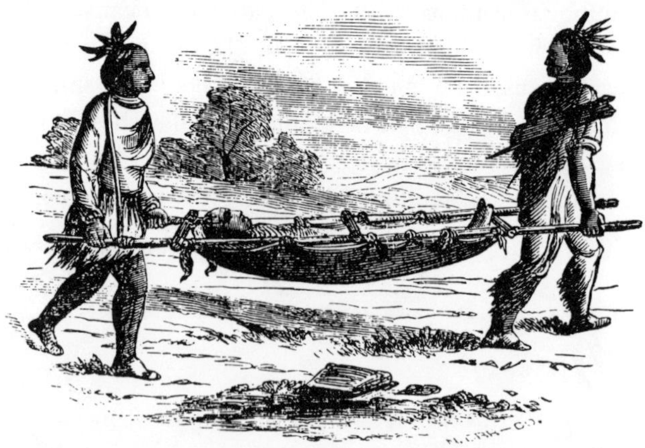

INDIAN HAND-LITTER. (From Galton.)

"American Indians carry their wounded companions by

this contrivance after a fight, and in a hurried retreat, for wonderful distances. A kind of wagon-top can easily be made to it with bent boughs and one spare blanket."

Dr. James R. Wood, of this city, Professor of Operative Surgery in Bellevue Medical College, has invented a very ingenious hand-litter. The poles being passed through loops on the side of the canvas, and the stretchers, or cross-bars, being made of steel, it can be very quickly rigged and unrigged, and can be rolled up into a very compact form. Several of the regiments recently organized have furnished themselves with these litters.

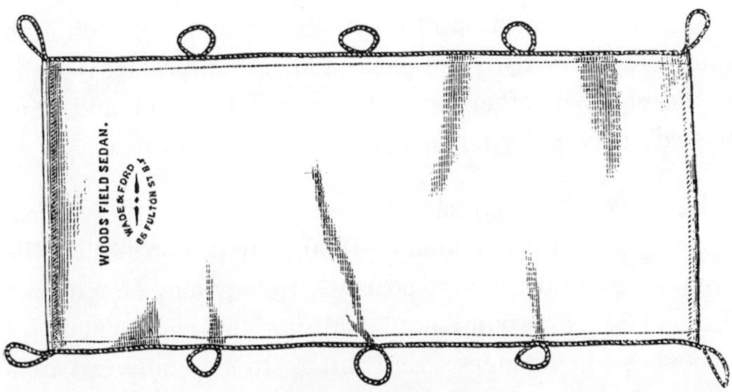

WOOD'S FIELD SEDAN.

SECTION II.—PANNIERS. In making long marches through a country where wheels are inadmissible, horses,

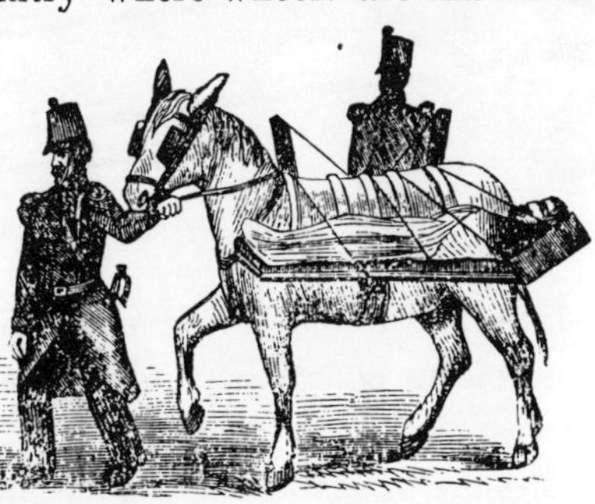

HORSE OR MULE PANNIER. (From Ballingall.)

mules, camels, etc., are occasionally put into requisition to convey the sick and wounded.

In the French service mules are employed for this purpose, fitted with panniers, one on each side of the animal. One of these panniers is intended to convey a soldier extended at length lying upon his back, and the opposite is constructed so as to receive a man in the sitting posture.

Baron Larrey describes, in the first volume of his Memoirs, a mode of conveyance for the sick adopted occasionally by the French army in Egypt, upon the backs of camels. "It consists of two large boxes or camel-trunks, fitted up as litters for the reception of the wounded, and slung, on each side of the animal, over a pack-saddle. The camel is made to kneel, as in other cases, to receive his load, and thus the sick may easily be placed in such a conveyance."

SECTION III.—HORSE-LITTERS. The Army Medical Board decided in January, 1860, "that horse-litters be prepared and furnished to posts where they may be required for service on ground not admitting the employment of two-wheeled carriages; said litters to be composed of a canvas bed similar to the present stretcher, and of two

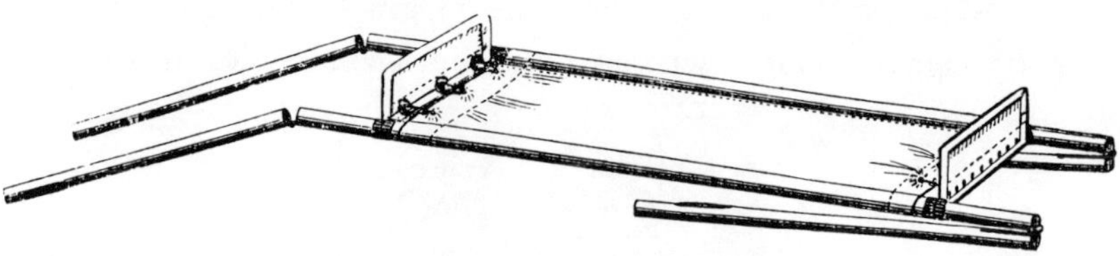

U. A. HORSE LITTER.

poles, each sixteen feet long, to be made in sections, with head and foot pieces constructed to act as stretchers to keep the poles asunder."

The side poles are of ash two and a half inches in diameter. The head and foot pieces are of canvas, stretched over strong iron wire, and are each nine inches in height. Width of canvas twenty-seven inches; length five feet ten inches.

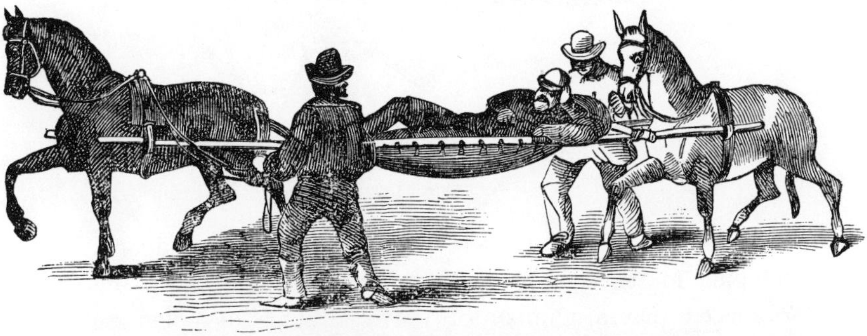

INDIAN HORSE OR MULE-LITTER. (From the Prairie Trav.)

SECTION IV.—WHEELED AMBULANCES. Where wheeled conveyances were necessary, the English and Americans have, until very lately, employed common spring wagons; but their inconvenience has at length led to the construction of others more suitable for the conveyance of the sick and wounded.

Of the various plans, Ballingall thinks that the carriage invented by Mr. Cherry is by far the most ingenious which he has seen. It is intended as a "hospital and commissariat" transport at the same time; and since the wounded need generally to be carried in a direction opposite to that in which the provisions, forage, etc., are to be carried, this may convey the latter to the army and bring back the former.

"It is a light single-horse cart, so constructed as to be readily adapted either to the carriage of stores and provisions, or to the conveyance of wounded men; for these two different purposes a great part of the frame-work is movable, and capable of being adapted to the object

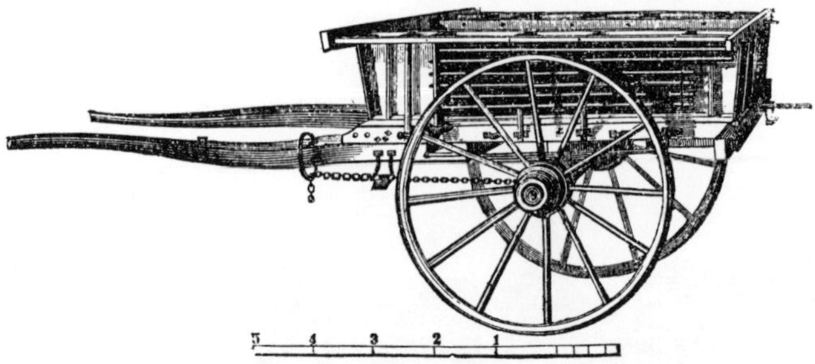

CHERRY'S CART.

required. In the state here represented, this carriage is adapted to the conveyance of provisions; and it will be observed that a number of movable spars or poles are stowed on the outside of the cart, which may in a few minutes be unpacked and placed upright round the framework, adapting it to the carriage of bulky articles of forage, such as hay or straw. Some of these spars, again, are fitted to be placed as ridgepoles on the top of the uprights,

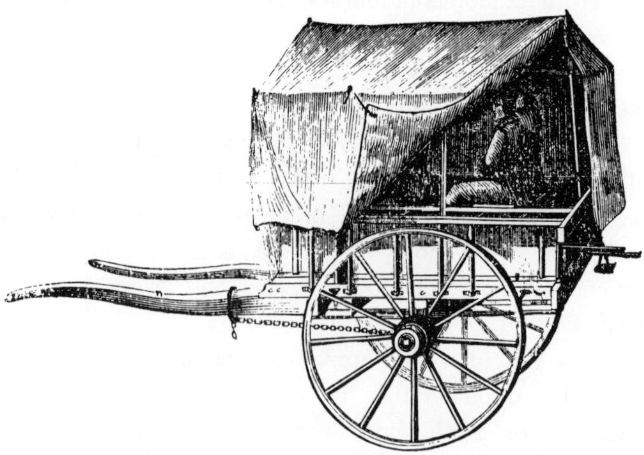

CHERRY'S CART.

for the purpose of supporting a canopy for the protection of the sick or wounded. It now becomes a most commodious sick-cart, capable of conveying one person lying at length on a board within, or four men sitting erect on seats, which are suspended from a rope running round the interior of the cart, and giving the advantage of its elasticity in addition to the springs. The seats, when not used for this purpose, form a movable part of the bottom of the cart, under which are boxes for containing the bearer and canopy when not wanted for their respective purposes. The most ingenious part of the contrivance is that by which the ordinary springs of a cart or other carriage may be protected from injury when carrying heavy loads, while at the same time it admits of their free use when light loads are carried. This is effected by two movable blocks sliding along the axle-tree; and which, by means of a lever connected with them, may either be moved outwards under the frame-work of the cart, so as to make its weight bear directly on the axle without injury to the springs, or, by turning the lever in an opposite direction, the blocks may be withdrawn from under the side-pieces of the cart into the hollow space formed by their thickness, and the springs thus again brought into action."

In January of last year, the United States Army Medical Board reported

"1. That ambulance transportation ought to be furnished for forty men per one thousand; twenty lying extended, and twenty sitting.

"2. That both two and four-wheeled ambulances are necessary for the hospital service.

"3. That a two-wheeled ambulance is the best for the conveyance of dangerously sick or dangerously wounded men.

"4. The Board being of opinion that both of the two-wheeled ambulances submitted to its inspection by Surgeon C. A. Finley and Assistant Surgeon R. H. Coolidge are well adapted to the purposes for which they were designed, and that their relative merits can only be determined by experiment, adopt both, and recommend that one of each pattern be sent to the respective military departments of Texas, New Mexico, Utah, California, and Oregon, and two of each pattern to Fort Leavenworth, and that they be placed in service at the scenes of Indian hostilities, and on marches across the plains, in order that their practical advantages may be ascertained.

"5. As the pattern of a four-wheeled ambulance designed by Surgeon Tripler, in the opinion of the Board, meets more fully the requirements of the service for the transportation of the slightly wounded, the slightly sick, and the convalescent, than any other pattern that has been submitted, the Board decide to adopt it, and recommend that three be constructed, and that one be sent to the Department of Texas, one to the Department of New Mexico, and one to Fort Leavenworth, in the Department of the West, for trial in active service.

"6. That of the two patterns of mattress-frames presented for examination by Assistant Surgeon Coolidge, the one without the box be adopted for trial.

"The Board then proceeded to the consideration of the amount and kind of transportation required for the sick and wounded, and for hospital supplies; the allowance of hospital stewards, cooks, and nurses, and also the nature and extent of tent accommodation, for troops on marches and in campaigns against Indians, and for a state of war with a civilized enemy.

"The following are the decisions and recommendations of the Board:

"1st. The Board recommend that the following amount and kind of transportation for the sick and wounded be provided for troops on marches and in campaigns against Indians:

"For commands of less than five companies, to each company, one two-wheeled ambulance.

"For a battalion of five companies, one four-wheeled and five two-wheeled ambulances.

"For a regiment, two four-wheeled and ten two-wheeled ambulances.

"2d. The Board, anxious to provide for the necessities and to secure the comfort of the sick and wounded soldiers to the fullest extent under all circumstances, recommend that the following schedule of transports for the sick and wounded and for hospital supplies, be adopted for a state of war with a civilized enemy:

"For commands of less than three companies, one two-wheeled transport cart for hospital supplies, and to each company one two-wheeled ambulance.

"For commands of more than three and less than five companies, two two-wheeled transport carts, and to each company one two-wheeled ambulance.

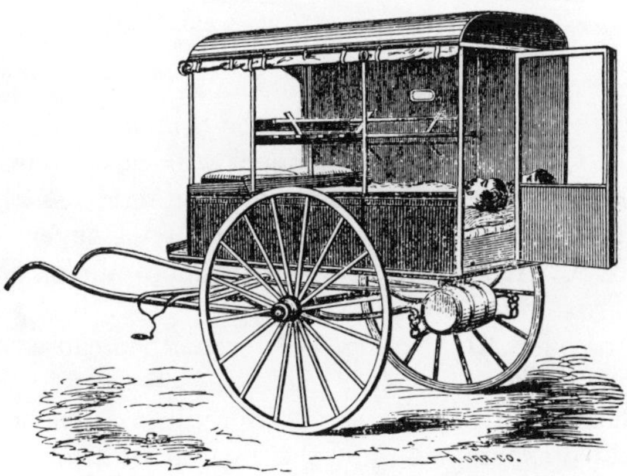

U. S. A. TWO-WHEELED AMBULANCE,

Designed by R. H. Coolidge, Surgeon, U. S. A.

"For a battalion of five companies, one four-wheeled ambulance, five two-wheeled ambulances, and two two-wheeled transport carts. For each additional company less than ten, one two-wheeled transport cart.

"For a regiment, two four-wheeled ambulances, ten two-wheeled ambulances, and four two-wheeled transport carts.

"That the transport carts be made after the model of the two-wheeled ambulances (their interior arrangement for the sick excepted), and to have solid board flooring to the body."

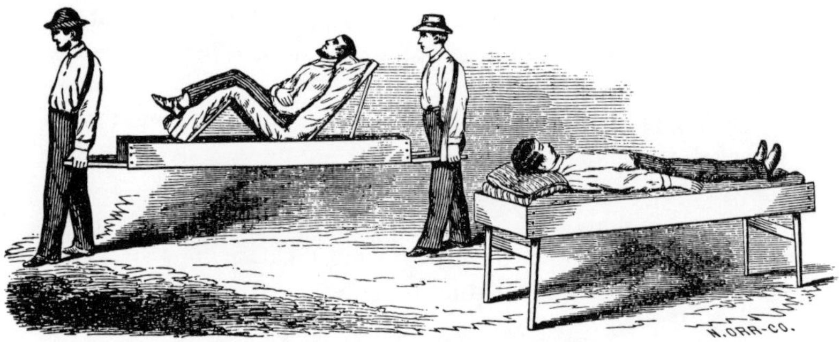

MATTRESSES FOR COOLIDGE'S AMBULANCE.

These recommendations were adopted, and the following order was immediately issued to the Secretary of War:

"The Quartermaster Department will cause ambulances of each pattern to be constructed without unnecessary delay, as follows: one at Philadelphia under the supervision of Surgeon C. A. Finley, one at Cincinnati under Surgeon C. S. Tripler, and one at Washington, D. C., under Assistant Surgeon R. H. Coolidge. He will then cause seven of each of the two-wheeled, and three of the four-wheeled ambulances to be constructed after these as models, and distributed as designated by the Board, for trial in active service according to the recommendation of the same, under direction of the several Department Commanders."

CHAPTER IX.

GUNSHOT WOUNDS.

GUNSHOT wounds are produced by a great variety of missiles, such as bullets, balls, buckshot, shrapnel, grape or canister, chain or bar shot, bombs, slugs, &c. These are all projected by the elastic power of gunpowder, and strike the body with great force, unless they are nearly spent. In their course from the weapon to their destination they describe a parabola; and smooth round balls, especially when the speed of their progress has been considerably arrested, revolve constantly upon their axes. It results in part from these two circumstances that a nearly spent round ball meeting with any obstacle, will readily deviate from its course. Hence those singular wounds in which a ball having entered at one point of the body is found exactly opposite, and it has not passed straight through but has made a partial circuit, leaving the contained viscera unharmed; or in which the ball has performed the entire circuit and appears at the very point at which it entered.

Hennen relates the case of a man in whom the ball, which struck the pomum Adami, was found lying in the orifice of its entrance, having gone completely around the neck. A similar case is reported by Prof. Malle in the 28th vol. of Amer. Jour. of Med. Sci. Oct. 1841.

In other cases, which seem equally singular, a man is killed instantly upon the field, and upon examination not a bruise, or wound, or fracture can be discovered. The soldiers say he was killed by the "wind" of a large ball, which has passed very near, but has not actually touched him. We know, however, that this is not the true explanation. He has been struck, probably, by a large and nearly spent ball, which may be said to have rolled over him, extinguishing life instantly by the concussion or shock; or it has been a side glance of one of these huge missiles.

The "shock" is not always fatal. Sometimes it is occasioned by a very slight injury; and this may happen even to the most courageous and intelligent, so that it cannot always be attributed to alarm. The soldier may be pale, tremulous, and unable to proceed, yet the wound which he has received may be trivial. On the other hand, even the most severe wounds may occasion no perceptible agitation.

Gunshot wounds are always contused, and often lacerated. Hence they are disposed to suppuration, sloughing, and secondary hæmorrhage. The primary hæmorrhage is, however, generally inconsiderable: and when it does occur, it is more often from a vein than from an artery. If a large arterial trunk has been only partially severed it bleeds more freely than when completely separated; and if severed by a ball passing with great rapidity it is more likely to bleed than if this has happened when the ball was moving slowly.

After a ball has penetrated the skin it generally meets with less resistance; and although it may be afterwards deflected from its straight course by muscles, tendons, fasciæ, or bones, yet it is pretty sure to penetrate deeply along the intermuscular or subcutaneous areolar tissue.

Arteries and nerves are frequently hit when lying in the track of a ball, but being thrust aside, are not always torn. These injuries are, however, liable always to be followed by secondary hæmorrhage, by tetanus, paralysis, or muscular atrophy.

Sometimes a round ball, striking a bone, is split into two or more fragments, some of which may pass entirely through, and others remain in the body.

Bullets now and then enter a certain distance, enveloped in a sac formed of the under clothing, and when the clothing is removed they are all withdrawn at the same time; in other cases they carry with them portions of the clothing, or other substances, which remain in the track, while the ball escapes at an opposite point. Slow balls drive in more pieces of clothes than balls in rapid motion.

At the point where a bullet makes its final lodgment, it is usually somewhat impacted, and entangled in the tissues. This is especially true of bullets which have been made irregular or rough by chewing them, as the Indians are known to do often; the conical bullet also becomes impacted, and is more difficult for this reason to remove.

The peculiar shape, great velocity, and rotary motion of conical balls impress certain characteristics upon the wounds which they inflict. They seldom deviate from a direct course after entering the body, nor do they often split; they produce great comminution of the bones; and when the range is short, the wound is generally smaller than that made by the round ball; but if the range is great, and the part thinly covered with soft tissues, then the wound is larger, especially at the point of exit; and more lacerated.

As an example of the curious freaks played by balls, we may mention a case which came under our own notice, in the year 1846:—A gentleman residing in Buffalo was assailed by a young midshipman, who discharged at him a pistol loaded with three bullets, and while standing about four paces distant. The gentleman's wallet lay in his pantaloons pocket, directly over the femoral artery, and on opening his wallet he found two of the bullets inside of it, lying loosely among some slips of paper. The third had glanced off, and lay upon the floor. Upon the skin, underneath the wallet, were two slight contusions, one on each side of the femoral artery.

Small shot, when they keep together, form a kind of bullet, but as they make a more lacerated and irregular wound, they are more fatal; but if they scatter they are less likely to kill.

Powder alone, with a wad, may perforate the tissues and kill, when the weapon is not distant.

Smooth, round balls, when embedded in the soft tissues, and not in contact with nerves, large arteries, joints, internal viscera, or other vital organs, do not always occasion much irritation, or cause even more than a temporary inconvenience. They sometimes become surrounded with a sort of fibrous cyst, and may remain for years without giving sufficient annoyance to point out their position. This is not true to the same extent of conical balls, of slugs, or of angular bodies of any character, or of balls which have penetrated the bones.

Dr. Kimball, of Mass., relates in the July No. for 1849, of the *New York Jour. of Med.*, the case of a man wounded in the hip by a ball, at Molino del Rey. The distinguished surgeon, Dr. Satterlee, who at that time had general charge of the hospitals, was unable to discover the ball, after a careful and thorough exploration. About three months later this man became epileptic, and the convulsive seizures continued during a period of five months, and until the ball was extracted by Dr. Kimball. It was found lying upon the great sciatic nerve. His recovery has been complete.

Treatment.—If practicable, and when the attempt is not attended with positive hazard, the ball or other missile should be at once removed. In order to accomplish this, a search must be instituted to determine its position. We should ascertain the relation which the weapon occupied to the person injured—its distance and direction—from which we may infer the depth to which the ball would be likely to penetrate, and its course under the skin. Ordinarily, if it has not passed entirely through, we should expect to find it upon the opposite side of the body, or of the limb, perhaps just beneath the integument. We should therefore feel for it with the finger here, and at many other points of the surface, near and remote; and not until we have exhausted other means ought we to introduce a probe along the track of the wound. We employ for this purpose the long probe, with an olive-shaped extremity, called the gunshot probe. (See Appendix A.)

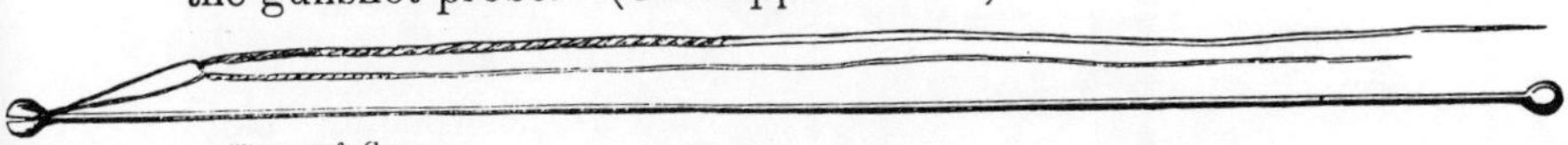
Tiemann & Co.

GUNSHOT PROBE.

A sound, or bougie, or flexible catheter, might answer in an emergency; but if the opening is sufficiently large, and the wound is not too deep, the finger is the best probe.

The limb should be placed, while conducting a probe

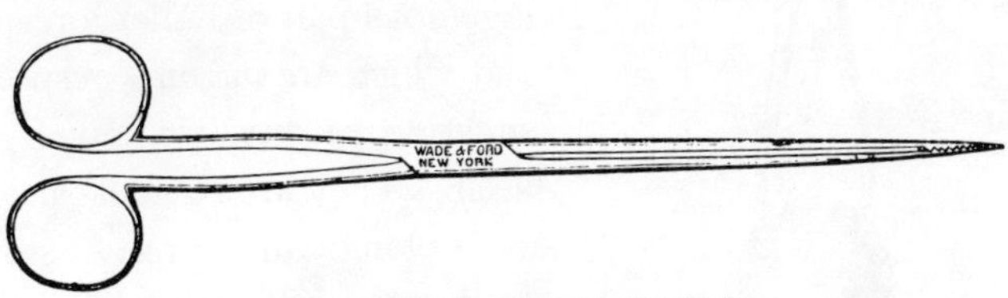

LONG, NARROW, BULLET FORCEPS.

along the track of the bullet, as nearly as possible in the same position as it was when the missile entered, otherwise, the change in the relative position of the integuments, muscles, &c., will render it difficult to follow the channel. Even a change of the muscles from an active to a passive condition, may be sufficient to close the canal.

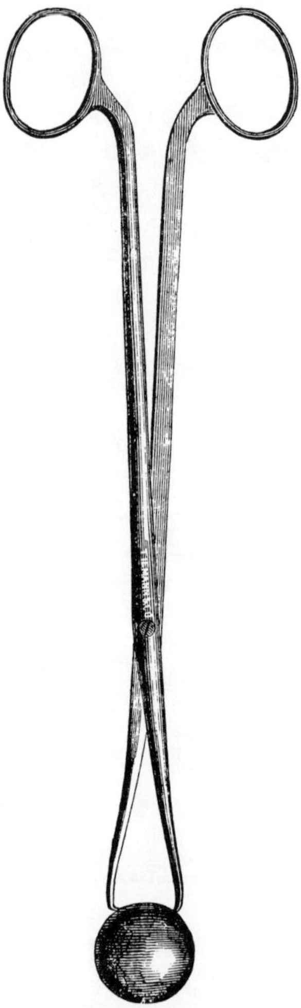

TIEMANN'S BULLET FORCEPS.

When the position of the ball is ascertained it may be cut upon and removed, or bullet forceps may be carried along the track, and the ball extracted through the same orifice at which it has entered.

Most of the bullet forceps are too clumsy to be of any service in deep and narrow channels. The best are the long slender forceps, serrated at the extremity; such as are represented in the woodcut, page 139.

George Tiemann & Co., the well-known instrument makers of 63 Chatham Street, New York, have invented a very ingenious pair of bullet forceps, and which are in some respects superior to any we have yet seen. They are so constructed with long and pretty stout teeth, set outward, like the incisors of a mouse, that they will seize upon a round leaden ball with great firmness, and even when only one quarter of the diameter is within the grasp of the instrument. These forceps would not be of much value, however, in the extraction of fragments of iron, or of any other hard metal.

When the ball has passed completely through, it is important sometimes to determine whether pieces of the clothing or other foreign substances have not been left in the track. A probe is always most easily admitted in the direction in which the ball has passed, the tissues being laid before the ball as grass falls before the wind. Generally we shall be able to determine the points of entrance and exit by their relative appearance. The opening where the ball has entered, is generally small, depressed, and contused; sometimes also blackened with powder; while the opening from which it has passed out is more often everted, lacerated, and larger. This is the general rule, yet it is liable to frequent exceptions.

Having removed the missile, it may become necessary, yet such is not often the fact, to take measures to arrest the hæmorrhage. If it is slight and proceeds from small vessels, cold or iced water may suffice; or if it is more considerable, we may sometimes resort to moderate compression; or, what is usually much better, to the persulphate of iron. This, diluted one half or more, may be injected into a deep wound by the syringe with which I have supplied my field case, or it may be laid undiluted on an open bleeding surface with a camel's hair brush. I have seen the persulphate of iron, injected into the cellular structure, produce erysipelatous inflammation; it is not, therefore, so innocuous as that it can be thrown of the full strength into the long track of a bullet, without some chance of its doing mischief. When the vessel is too large for the bleeding to be restrained by these means, we must at once proceed to tie the artery from which the hæmorrhage proceeds—in the wound if we can—and perhaps that can be done by laying it freely open; but if we cannot reach it here we must cut down and tie above.

If a tourniquet becomes necessary, we prefer the ordinary screw tourniquet, invented by J. L. Petit.

In an emergency we may employ as a substitute the simple field tourniquet, composed of a strap and buckle, either with or without a pad; or a simple cord, twisting it tightly with a stick, a pistol, or any short weapon. (See App. B.)

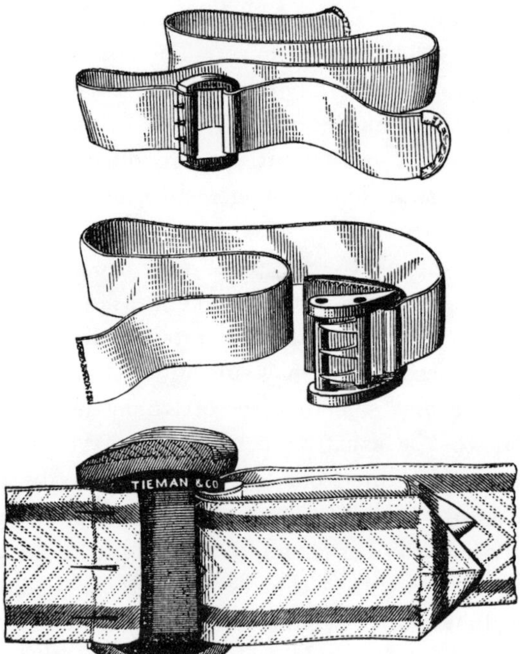

FIELD TOURNIQUETS.

Ordinarily no other treatment or dressing is necessary for a gunshot wound, than to lay upon it a piece of lint saturated with cool or cold water. Sometimes, however, the condition of the parts demands that the applications should be warm, so as to encourage the return of its vitality.

Baudens, who served in the Crimea, recommends ice, as a first application. The English surgeons in the same expedition employed the water dressings to the exclusion of almost everything else; but Surgeon McLeod thinks that "when inflammation and suppuration are present, *hot* applications will always be found of most good."

If water irrigations are employed, a very simple method is to bore with a gimlet a hole in the side of a pail, near the bottom, but not so near as that the dirt which settles in the pail will escape through the hole. Insert into the opening a piece of a goose quill, and draw through this a few threads of common candle wicking. Placing the pail upon a table, or suspending it above the limb, the candle wicking terminating upon the piece of patent lint with which the wounded member is covered, the water diffuses itself gently and equally over the whole surface.

At a little later period the lotions may be slightly medicated with chloride of soda or of lime, as an antiseptic.

The practice of crowding tents into gunshot wounds, is, we are happy to say, nearly abandoned at the present day.

If sloughing takes place, yeast or charcoal poultices will be necessary.

From about the fifth to the twelfth or fifteenth day, and sometimes for a longer period, the limb ought to be kept very quiet, and unusual care taken in removing the dressings, lest a secondary hæmorrhage should be occasioned.

If secondary hæmorrhage does actually occur to such an extent as to cause alarm, and which cannot be arrested by posture, by moderate pressure, by cold applications, or by the persulphate of iron, no time ought to be lost in securing the bleeding vessel above the wound. It is seldom possible to arrest such hæmorrhages by plugging or by tying the vessel within the wound.

In relation to the treatment of gunshot wounds with simple water dressings, I shall take the liberty of quoting somewhat at length from a treatise written by Alphonse Amussat, at Paris, in 1851, and which I translated the same year. (Buffalo Med. Jour., 1851. Also published in the form of an octavo volume.)

"In 1786, Lombard published in his *Opuscules de Chirurgie* a very remarkable article, in which he established the value of a therapeutic agent until then too much neglected, and opened a new road which soon had to be followed by the surgeons of the French armies during the great wars of the revolution, and of the empire. This work, entitled 'Summary of the properties of simple water, employed as a topical application in the cure of surgical maladies,' is divided into two parts: in the first, he treats of the properties and advantages of cold water; while he devotes the second to the consideration of tepid water and to an examination of the affections and temperaments which demand the use of tepid rather than cold water, and the reverse.

"Percy being at Strasbourg in 1785, as surgeon-major of the regiment of Berry, had an opportunity of seeing the results obtained by Lombard from simple water dressings upon some soldiers wounded in a trial of ordnance. A quick observer, he comprehended immediately all the advantages of this mode of treatment upon the field of battle. We may judge of his opinions by the following passages, copied from his article entitled 'water,' in the 'Dictionary of Medical Sciences;' an article which contains in germ nearly all the applications of water which have been made since in the treatment of surgical affections, even irrigations.

"'Among the kind of miracles,' says he, 'which I have seen wrought by water in wounds from fire-arms, I will instance the cure of nearly sixty young volunteers of a battalion called "Louvre," which having left Paris on the first day of December 1792, was ordered on Christmas-day to the assault upon Montagne Verte, near Treves. The enemy placed upon a height, made upon the battalion a well sustained fire, and most of these young men were wounded in their feet. Many were taken to the military hospital of Sarrelouis, of whom only a few could be saved without amputation. The others remained in the convent of Consarrebruck, with two German surgeons, who were charged with their care. By my advice, and *perhaps in default of other remedies*, the attendants bathed their feet incessantly, and showered them with water moderately cool, covering their wounds with compresses constantly moistened with the same. No other dressings were used, and I attest that only four died, of whom two died of adynamic fever, which disturbed and interrupted the treatment of the wounds with water; one of colliquative diarrhea, and the fourth of trismus. All the others recovered rapidly; several had not even anchylosis, although their feet had been traversed in every direction, complicated with tearing of tendons, aponeuroses, and ligaments, and with splintering of the bones, sometimes of the tarsus, sometimes of the metatarsus.'

"Larrey relates in the following manner the advantages which he derived from the use of water in the campaign in Egypt.

"'One would be astonished without doubt, to learn that with a few sea biscuit, a little good water which was carried with each wounded man, and *by the use of brackish water only for their dressings*, a very great number of these individuals, suffering under severe wounds of the head, of the breast, of the abdomen, or deprived of some of their limbs, crossed the deserts which separate Syria from Egypt, a distance of about sixty leagues, without any accident, and with so much benefit, that most of them found themselves cured when they reached this latter country.'

"Briot, a very distinguished military surgeon, is much

pleased with the employment of water, which he regards as *le vulneraire par excellence*, in the dressing of wounds received upon the field of battle.

"'The general method of dressing which we employed,' says he, 'consisted in doing nothing without a motive. We use with success, and almost always to the accomplishment of perfect cures, *cold water* in wounds made by small-arms; also in cases of stupor, in wounds of tendons, of aponeuroses, of capsules and of membranes; and *tepid water* in those made by fire-arms and which were suppurating.'

"The most notable cases of success resulting from the use of water in gunshot wounds are unquestionably those reported by Dr. Treille, after the battle of Baylen.

"'I obtained, seven years ago, the most happy effects from the indiscriminate application of pure water upon every variety of gunshot wounds.

"A very extraordinary circumstance compelled me to employ this means alone. I confess that at first I was not without some solicitude as to the results, but I was quickly reassured by my success. The facts were thus: After the battle of Baylen (Andalusia), I remained upon the field the only surgeon to take care of five hundred wounded. Deprived of all medicines, I had all the wounds washed with pure water. I continued my dressings in this way during twenty-one days that we remained upon the field of battle, receiving nothing from without but some linen and provisions. As it would have been impossible for me alone to dress five hundred wounded, I arranged them in three sections and dressed one section each day, and they dressed themselves the two other days.

"'Only seven or eight wounds became gangrenous, and I had but two cases of tetanus.

"'When attention is given to the circumstances in which I was placed, it will be apparent what we ought to think of simple water in the treatment of recent wounds. Here were five hundred wounded lying upon the ground from the nineteenth of June to the tenth of July (1808), under the broiling sun of Andalusia, having nothing whatever for shade but the thin branches of olive trees, deprived of the consolatory hope of ever again seeing their own country, and given up to the mercy of the inhabitants of Sierra-Morena, who were all in arms and highly exasperated.

"'In a word, the moral as well as the physical was but little favorable to the treatment of wounds; I have shown you, nevertheless, what was my success."

"'By cold water,' says Guthrie, 'the inflammation is in certain cases entirely prevented, in many greatly controlled, and in almost all much subdued, while the suppurative process is not sufficiently impeded to prevent the subsequent action of granulation. In all simple cases of gunshot wounds, that is to say wounds which implicate only the soft parts, in persons of a healthy constitution, a little lint dipped in oil, or on which some ointment has been spread, is the best application in the first instance to prevent irritation: supporting the whole with two strips of adhesive plaster laid across. A compress or folds of linen wetted with water are then to be applied over it, and to be kept constantly wet and cold, even by the use of ice, if it can be obtained, and it be found comfortable to the patient.'

"And a little farther on,

"'Cold water is not an infallible remedy; its use is not even always advantageous: there are many persons with whom cold applications do not agree; there are more with whom they disagree after a certain period, and in these two cases they should not be persisted in. Cold does no good at any stage of inflammation, when the sensation produced by the first application is disagreeable to the patient, and when it does not soothe; for if it produces a sensation of shivering, or any other uncomfortable feeling; if it causes a stiffness in the part, it is doing harm, and if we change the treatment and cause a genial sensation of warmth in the limb, it will not only prove more comfortable, but be found actually advantageous. This happens in general at the period of the commencement of suppuration; and in such cases cold prevents the complete effect of the suppurative action, which heat favors. Fomentations are then excellent.'

"Prof. V. Kern, of Vienna, published in 1809 a work in which he recommends tepid water in the treatment of wounds.

"Among the authors who have written upon this subject we will mention, in France, MM. Rouboud, Mauricheau-Beaupre, Laurent, Tanchou, Cloquet, Serre (of Uzes), Marjolin, Blandin, etc.; in England, Samuel Cooper; in Germany, Dzondi, professor at Halle, Rust, etc.; Mayor, of Lausanne.

"We should also mention in a particular manner, Sanson, who writes thus in his article upon 'Water' in the 'Dictionary of Practical Medicine and Surgery,' published in 1831:

"'With water,' says he, 'I have seen cured by first intention contused wounds, accompanied with more or less laceration and stretching of the parts; I have been able to save most persons upon whom I have practised amputation, or other grave operations, from the fever called traumatic; indeed I have been able to cure, without amputation, and even without active inflammation or copious suppuration, many persons having fractured limbs complicated with wounds and projection of the fragments.'

"The eulogium which Sanson bestows upon water is based upon extensive experience, and it acquires more value when it is known with what cautious reserve this expert surgeon adopts all surgical innovations.

"From this historical glance we see that the use of water in surgery has made great advances since the publication of the work of Lombard. During the wars of the Revolution and of the Empire, necessity often compelled surgeons to resort to it, and it is surprising that, seeing the success which att nded their practice, it has not come to be generally adopted. Fomentations and effusions, the only methods then employed, although very simple in their application, really efficacious, and possessed of all the advantages of cataplasms without their inconveniences, still left much to be desired.

"M. Baudens, ever partial to the traditions of military surgery, and to the principles of Lombard, of Percy, of Larrey, of Treille, and of Guthrie, thus speaks in his 'Treatise upon Gunshot Wounds,' in relation to his own practice since the commencement of the African campaign:

"'The dressings of wounds should be as mild as possible; such as perforated linen smeared with cerate, lint, compresses, and rollers. These dressings should be wet with cold water constantly for several days.'

"Since then M. Baudens has always professed the same doctrines that he taught in his book; he has even gone farther, for he employs now ice and refrigerant mixtures with success. But we must not forget that besides great experience in the use of this therapeutic means, the surgeon of Val-de-Grace had generally *only strong and robust young men to treat,* and we shall understand how he could be so successful with an agent at once so powerful, and, as we think, so dangerous.

"In 1839, our worthy *confrère,* M. Lacorbiere, issued his learned 'Treatise upon Cold,' employed both externally and internally 'as a hygienic, medical, and surgical agent,' In this work, the most complete which our science possesses upon this subject, the author sustains with great justness of argument, supported by numerous facts, all the advantages which had been claimed for cold water in surgical affections. In a letter addressed to M. Lacorbiere, and published in his work, M. Alquie declares in these words his opinion upon the use of water:—

"'I have under a multitude of circumstances,' says he, 'derived advantages, *almost marvellous,* from the action of cold water, and from ice in cases of severe traumatic lesions. In 1823, when I directed the medico-chirurgical service of the hospital of Perthus, I attributed to this means the cure of several gun-shot wounds situated in the feet and hands. In the case of a drummer of the eighth regiment of voltigeurs, whose right foot had been traversed by a ball, breaking the first cuneiforme and producing great disturbance of the parts, I could only avoid serious accidents by the diligent application of cold water to the wounded member.

"'Especially in large contused wounds has this means been useful. When I was surgeon-major of the sixth regiment of dragoons, a captain of this regiment, M. David, received at Pontivy a kick from a horse upon the middle of his right leg. A large wound, four inches in length, resulted from the tearing of the inner half of the gemellus and the integuments. The periosteum along a portion of the tibia had been scratched by the iron, which had made an indentation in the inner side of the bone; it was a horrible wound! Ice water applied continuously during sixty hours, prevented completely all immoderate inflammatory action, and this extensive solution of continuity united almost without suppuration. It appeared that we had the power to regulate the inflammation precisely to the condition necessary for re-union.'

"I could cite similar cases which occurred among the dragoons of the sixth regiment, and several others at the hospital of Toulon and of Alger.

"In 1841, Mathias Mayor, in his 'Surgery Simplified,' writes thus:—'Water has been invoked and proclaimed in every age and by the greatest surgeons, as the most important agent in the treatment of most surgical affections, and as the means, *par excellence*, to favor the efforts of nature. It is to be regretted that this opinion, so prevalent among surgeons and physicians, has had so little influence with the people, and especially with military men.

"In 1842, M. Malgaigne presented to the concours of the surgical clinique of the Faculty of Medicine of Paris, a thesis upon 'irrigation in surgical affections.' This truly excellent work winds up with the following conclusions:

" 'First, cold irrigations are an excellent antiphlogistic when employed in superficial wounds or inflammations; but even then they are not infallible, whilst in deeper wounds and inflammations they only mask the symptoms, and ought to be rejected.

" 'Second, continued irrigations are only suitable for the hands and feet, and perhaps the forearm, but my facts are not sufficient upon this last point to decide; and even in these regions recourse should not be had to them except in the most severe cases. I give them an almost absolute preference in gun-shot wounds, but for other wounds I prefer intermittent irrigations.

" 'Third, in all cases the parts undergoing irrigation should be carefully covered with compresses, so as to exclude the air.

" 'Fourth, simple water appears preferable for continued irrigations, but for intermittent irrigations I choose *eau blanche* (plumbi diacetas, &c.) in cases of wounds, and a solution of sulphate of copper or wine in cases where no wound exists.

" 'Fifth, the temperature must *vary* according to the sensations experienced by the patient when the water is first applied: and in all cases we must abridge the duration of the irrigations as much as possible.'

"I believe with M. Malgaigne, that irrigations are not absolutely infallible any more than other means employed in surgery; but, with the numerous facts which I possess of lesions located in almost every part of the body, forearm, leg, and knee, I cannot agree with him in the limits which he has placed upon its use. As to the duration of the irrigations, I think, where a moderate temperature is suitable, they may be continued a long time with advantage, and I am reminded among others, of a case, which I will soon publish, where a cure was effected of a severe wound of the leg, by irrigations of water at a temperature of 20° C. (68° F.) continued more than two months.

Gunshot wounds of the head are generally fatal, whether the ball passes entirely through or remains within the skull, and this is especially true of gunshot wounds of the anterior half and base of the brain. Yet the exceptions to this rule are numerous. One of the most extraordinary cases of recovery upon record, probably, is that of the man Gage, who was shot through the head with a tamping iron, three feet seven inches in length, one inch and a quarter in diameter at its largest end, and weighing thirteen pounds and a quarter.

The accident occurred in 1848, and Dr. Harlow, of Cavendich, Vermont, in whose practice the case occurred, described the wound as commencing just anterior to the ramus of the inferior maxillary bone of the left side, taking a direction upward and backward toward the median line, passing through the left anterior lobe of the cerebrum, and making its exit at the junction of the coronal and sagittal sutures; lacerating the longitudinal sinus; extensively fracturing the frontal and parietal bones; breaking up a large portion of the brain, and protruding the globe of the left eye from its socket by nearly one-half its diameter.

In 1860 this man was still living, and in the enjoyment of good health, with no impairment whatever of his mental faculties.

Not a few examples also are upon record where foreign bodies having entered the brain, have remained in this situation months and years without causing death. Larrey mentions that a portion of the blade of a javelin remained in the brain fourteen years, and was then extracted successfully; and Dr. Trumbull speaks of a child in whose brain remained a piece of iron spindle three inches in length, for a period of eight years, but who finally died from the effects of the removal.

In Chelius's Surgery will be found an account of several more of these curious cases; and in a Philadelphia journal for November, 1858, we read the following:

"A man named Courshan was yesterday convicted in the court of Quarter Sessions of an assault and battery, with intent to kill. This case is somewhat extraordinary. A number of colored men got into a street brawl about a woman, and one of them fired a pistol at one of the party, a sailor. The slug from the pistol pierced the skull of the sailor and buried itself deep in his brain. The wounded man was taken to the hospital, where his wound was dressed without the ball being extracted, and the sufferer was left to die. But he did not die. In course of time he recovered, and he has now actually gone to sea with a slug in his brain. 'Time was that when the brain was out the man would die,' and it has hitherto been considered rather a hazardous experiment to drill a man's head with a pistol ball. The case we refer to has proved an exception to the established rules."

But these examples only demonstrate the extraordinary resources of nature, and are not to be regarded as constituting a correct basis for prognosis.

When a bullet has entered the skull and not passed completely through, it cannot generally be found. The force which was sufficient to penetrate the bone has in most cases proved sufficient also to lodge the missile quite or nearly upon the opposite side. It is generally impracticable therefore to reach it with the probe. Moreover, it is exceedingly unsafe to attempt to enter a probe along the track of a wound of the brain, at least to any considerable depth, owing to the softness of the natural structure of the brain, and the consequent difficulty of determining whether the probe is entering the channel made by the missile, or the brain itself. The finger ought always to be used instead of the probe, if the opening is sufficiently large for its admission.

Dr. Hann, of the United States Army, relates a case in which the ball was found resting upon the dura mater directly under the wound in the skull. He trephined the man, removed the ball, and the recovery was complete.—*Am. Jour. M.S.*, April, 1841.

If the bullet is found, it cannot generally be extracted through the same opening in the skull at which it has entered; and the trephine must be applied to render the opening sufficiently large to admit the forceps. When found, no pains should be spared to accomplish its extraction.

Openings through the skull made by large conical balls are generally more irregular and larger than those made by round balls, and afford therefore a better opportunity for their extraction.

We ought to take especial pains to remove all the small fragments of bone which are so generally found broken off from the internal plate after these accidents.

The subsequent treatment consists in the application of a piece of lint wetted with cold water; rest, cathartics, low diet, bleeding, etc. In short, the treatment must be rigidly antiphlogistic, and this general plan needs to be pursued, in most cases, for a long time, since the patient is for many weeks liable to the recurrence or sudden accession of inflammation. The head should remain constantly in an elevated position.

If fragments of bone subsequently exfoliate, they must be removed as soon as their separation is complete.

The concussion occasioned by a bullet is frequently slight and temporary. When severe, it must be treated by rest and a somewhat expectant plan until reaction occurs, after which cathartics and low diet may be necessary.

Wounds of the thorax, whether gunshot or produced by sword or bayonet thrust, are not, as a class, so fatal as wounds of the head. If the bullet enters the heart or any of the larger vessels the wound is fatal; but sometimes the wounded man owes his safety to the resiliency of the ribs, in consequence of which the ball is turned aside and does not enter the chest at all; or, having entered, it passes between the lungs, through the mediastinal spaces; or penetrating the lungs, air is admitted into the pleural cavity, and to a greater or less extent the wounded lobe collapses, thus preventing in some degree the hæmorrhage which otherwise would have occurred. However this may be, it is certain that a considerable number of those who receive chest wounds, and in which the missile passes entirely through, recover. The records of surgery abound with examples of this kind. On the 17th of April, 1855, Michael Shaler was shot through his right lung, the ball, having entered in front between the fifth and sixth ribs and passed entirely out from the opposite side of his chest, was found in his shirt. I saw him immediately after the accident. He was lying on his back; he was pale, and his breathing somewhat embarrassed; only a small amount of blood was expectorated. On the first day of the following September I found him in perfect health. He had not been under my care after the first day, and I cannot speak of the treatment.

I have also met with a number of penetrating wounds of the thorax produced by sharp, pointed instruments, all of which, I think, except one have resulted in complete recovery.

Dr. Mills, surgeon in the United States Army, has mentioned to me that he had seen a soldier in the Florida war, attempting to desert, shot throught the right lung with a carbine ball, and who recovered in ten days without the occurrence of suppuration.

Dr. Amasa Trowbridge of Watertown, United States surgeon in the war of 1812, writes to me as follows: "Major Trimble, at the sortie made upon the British batteries near Fort Erie, received a wound by a musket ball through the right portion of the thorax; it entered and divided the fifth rib near its cartilaginous extremity, passed through the lung and divided the same rib near its curvature towards the spine, and passed out. He was engaged at the time in carrying one of the enemy's block-houses. Blood flowed freely from his mouth, and external wounds; respiration was at times nearly suspended, with feeble pulse and cold extremities. I shall not be able to give a particular history of his treatment, but I well remember that but little hope of his recovery was entertained, until the fifth day after receiving the wound. From the time of the accident to this period, bleeding from the external wound gradually subsided, but the prostration of the system was great from the first. Reaction, however, took place, and so steady and continued was it, that he was bled six times within twenty days. It was to the repeated bleedings, together with the kind care of his friend Colonel McRea, who remained with him constantly, that I ascribed his final recovery. After the close of the war he distinguished himself in the councils of this state (Ohio), and was employed by the general government to transact important business with some of the western tribes of Indians. He was elected member of the United States Senate in 1822. His fatigue and exposure at the West, the previous season, had aggravated an affection of the lungs, which proved fatal a few days after his arrival in Washington."

Dr. D. C. Peters, Assistant Surgeon, United States Army, reports in the November Number for 1860 of the New York Medical Times, a case of complete recovery after a wound through the left breast, made by a "slug" discharged from a Sharpe's carbine, the track of the wound being very near the heart.

The following letter from Dr. Wright of the United States Army, giving an account of the case of General Shields, who was shot through the chest at Cerro Gordo, will be found exceedingly pertinent and of remarkable interest.

"FORT LEAVENWORTH, *March* 10*th*, 1861.

"MY DEAR SIR:—At the request of our mutual friend, Surgeon M. Mills of the army, I am induced to send you the following brief and very imperfect report of the case of General Shields, whose recovery has been the subject of much comment and marvel, in and out of the army.

"The necessities of the service having disconnected me with the case, twelve hours after the infliction of the wound, I regret that I am unable to delineate the minute features of its history, from day to day, up to the period of the General's restoration to duty: but what I regret still more is, that having lost the notes I took of the case, I am forced to rely on my memory alone, for the partial facts I communicate.

"General Shields, in command of his Brigade, at the battle of Cerro Gordo, on the 18th of April, 1847, was stricken down by canister shot, from one of the Mexican batteries, in front of which his brigade was drawn up. I saw the General perhaps fifteen or twenty minutes after his fall. He was lying on his back. His objective condition was as follows:—External surface of the body almost exsanguine; animal powers prostrate; organic forces very feeble; pulse frequent and almost imperceptible at the wrist; respiration hurried and anxious; voice inarticulate above a whisper, and the blood was flowing profusely from both orifices of the wound.

"On examination, I found that the missile (presumed from the character and dimensions of the wound, to be a canister shot) had penetrated between the fourth and fifth ribs of the right side, an inch and a half or two inches from the sternum, and had emerged between the sixth and seventh ribs of the same side, about an inch or little more from their junction with the vertebræ. I proceeded of course at once to stanch the bleeding wounds, as the first and most important indication to be fulfilled. This was done by the application of dry lint, thrust within the orifices, and secured by compress and roller. The case did not seem to demand further interference, except a resort to cautious stimulation, to the extent necessary to sustain the sinking powers of life, from loss of blood. Up to the completion of the dressing, the General was literally silent, and I refrained from communicating to him, uninvited, the prognosis I had formed: then, however, with his finger he beckoned me to apply my ear to his mouth, when he said in a faint voice, 'I know my condition is a most dangerous one, and suppose I must die:—tell me candidly your opinion, and do not deceive me.' I said in substance, 'I will not deceive you, General. Your condition is a most critical one, but for your slight encouragement, I will inform you that the annals of surgery furnish many instances to prove, and my own experience in this war has taught me, that gun-shot wounds of the chest, even though the substance of the lungs may have been transfixed, are not necessarily fatal.' I was glad to find the General apparently satisfied with my response, inasmuch as if he had had the strength and the will to catechise me further on the subject, I would have been forced to admit that neither my reading nor experience furnished any case essentially parallel to his, where recovery ensued.

"General Shields remained on the battle-field from about ten o'clock A. M., when I first saw him, until near sun-down, when he was carried to a house on the road-side, near the foot of Telegraph Hill, where he remained under the care of Surgeon McMillan of the volunteer corps, for several weeks, when he was transported on a litter to Jalapa. Here he recovered, in time to join the army on its march to the valley of Mexico, where, in several of the battles, he was again distinguished for his intrepid gallantry and daring courage: in one of which, he received a severe wound of the fore-arm, from an escopet ball.

"As I intimated above, I was compelled to proceed with the army in its onward march towards the Mexican Capital, the day after the battle, and as General Shields was not in condition to admit of removal from Cerro Gordo, I was obliged to relinquish the charge of his case. Fortunately he fell into competent hands, and under the skilful care of Surgeon McMillan, he recovered, and is a living illustration of the wisdom of the maxim, 'Nil desperandum.'

"Fortunately for General Shields the result of the case did not admit of a post-mortem examination, to reveal the course of the missile, or the structures which it penetrated in its passage. To my mind it is abundantly evident that entering between the ribs in front, it passed through both pleuræ, and of course through the substance of the right lung (middle lobe), and emerged between the sixth and seventh ribs.

"Having lost sight of Surgeon McMillan since the Mexican war, I am unable to avail myself of his memoranda, and more intimate knowledge of the case, in its progress towards recovery. My impression is that no hæmorrhage from the external wounds occurred after the first dressing, and that no untoward event happened, requiring more than slight interference with the efforts of the vis medicatrix. At Jalapa, during the General's convalescence, some dulness was perceptible on percussion, and though, if I remember rightly, the respiratory murmur was not wholly abolished *anywhere*, as indicated by the ear, it was sensibly modified, and diminished in the region of the wound.

"I met the General frequently in Mexico, after his recovery, and came with him to the coast. I am not aware that he suffers any impairment of health, or constitutional vigor, which can be in any way traced to the terrific wound he received at Cerro Gordo.

"Reiterating my apology for the imperfect character of this report,

"I am, sir, very repectfully, your obedient servant,

"J. J. B. WRIGHT, Surgeon U.S.A."

The prognosis is, of course, much less favorable when the ball has lodged within the cavity of the thorax, and cannot be found or extracted. McLeod says, that of thirty-three cases, in which the ball lodged in the chest, or appeared to lodge, thirty-one died. It is said, however, that the *post mortem* of the body of Prince Jerome led to the discovery of a ball which had remained in his chest after a duel which he fought in his youth, with a brother of Marshal Davoust.

The same remark made in relation to gunshot wounds of the head, applies to similar wounds of the chest, namely, that the bullet is seldom found near the orifice, but usually on the opposite side, or to a considerable depth in the substance of the lungs; but if it has entered the lung in any degree the immediate collapse of that portion will so change its relation to the external orifice that the bullet is not likely to be found. Even when it has gone no deeper than the pleura, the same difficulty must be experienced in the search, as it will fall to some other part of the pleural cavity.

The examination will therefore consist, generally, in a limited exploration of the track of the wound, especially with a view to determine whether any pieces of clothing have been carried in, and in an inspection, or careful digital manipulation of the opposite side of the thorax. Auscultation is only serviceable at a later period, nor can it be practised satisfactorily during the agitation usually consequent upon such an injury. Bloody expectoration furnishes almost positive evidence that the structure of the lungs is penetrated. The absence of this sign, however, is not proof so positive that the lungs have not been penetrated.

The treatment consists in covering the wound with a pledget of lint, saturated with cool water, the employment of sedatives, and of antiphlogistics. The patient must be requested to lie upon the wounded side, or in such a position as that the orifice shall be depending, unless the wound is on the front of the chest. Often this is impracticable, certain positions being more painful and interfering more with the respiration than others. We have no choice then but to leave the patient to adopt that position which he finds most comfortable.

Few, comparatively, die of hemorrhage after being wounded in the chest, unless the heart or some large blood-vessel has been opened: more die of the subsequent inflammation, and a certain proportion, at a still later period, succumb to abscesses, or to other chronic maladies of the thoracic viscera.

When emphysema occurs, recognised by the peculiar crepitation produced by the presence of air in the cellular tissue, the external wound should be rendered as free as possible; and when the emphysema is extensive, small incisions, here and there, in the subcutaneous cellular tissue may become necessary. We must say, however, that we have seen many cases of emphysema occasioned by broken ribs, and wounds in the chest, in some of which the emphysema has extended over more than half the body, yet it has never resulted in death, or even seemed to endanger life by any degree of embarrassment to the respiration. Nor have we ever found it necessary to scarify the skin to afford relief. The extravasation of air has in all cases ceased spontaneously; and after the lapse of periods varying from one to six or seven weeks, it has been completely absorbed without any surgical or therapeutical aid.

If one of the intercostal arteries has been wounded it should be held by the finger and pressed against the rib until it ceases to bleed, or with the aid of a pair of curved forceps and a needle it must be tied.

If wounds of the chest have acquired a certain degree of notoriety from the number of recoveries which have taken place, wounds of the belly are no less remarkable for the numbers who die. Wounds of the liver and spleen, or of any of the large blood-vessels contained within the abdomen, generally cause death from hemorrhage very quickly. A wound of the superficial portion of the liver is, however, not always fatal. Wounds of the other viscera result in death generally by the production of inflammation.

Bullets entering the belly cannot generally be extracted unless they are on the opposite side, and can be felt from that point: first, because we do not know where to search for them, and second, because the search is in itself attended with the most imminent hazard to the life of the patient.

In the natural condition of the parts, that portion of the peritoneum which covers the intestines is in absolute contact everywhere with that portion which lines the walls of the abdomen. When a bullet or a bayonet has entered the belly, the intestines or stomach may have been wounded, but it is by no means certain that they have not escaped; or if they have been actually penetrated, there still remains some ground for hope that their contents have not found their way into the cavity of the peritoneum. If they have not, the danger is much lessened, and it will be our object now to prevent this extravasation as far as possible. If we were to lay open the external wound in order to find the ball, or to ascertain the condition of the viscera, such extravasations would probably occur; or if we were even to introduce a probe, air would be admitted from without, and the same thing would happen.

To give to our patient, therefore, the best chance of recovery, we have to pursue an almost expectant plan. He must be laid upon his back, with his body a little flexed; a piece of adhesive plaster should be made to close the wound completely; he should be allowed no drink or food for several hours, unless it be a little ice-water or small pieces of ice at intervals. Everything received into the stomach, however bland, is apt to excite peristaltic motion, and to endanger extravasation; no cathartic or even enema; he should not be permitted to turn to the right or to the left in bed, or get up for any reason whatever. If he suffers much pain, opiates and poultices may be necessary; and eventually leeches or the lancet may be demanded.

After wounds of the bladder, a flexible catheter must be kept in the urethra, and if possible, counter-openings made through which the extravasated urine may escape.

If the bladder was full at the time of the receipt of the injury, death is pretty certain to follow in a few days; and the danger is much increased when the wound penetrates the peritoneal covering of the bladder.

Dr. N. S. Jarvis, Surgeon in the United States Army, reports, in the March number for 1847, of the American Medical Journal, three cases of gunshot wounds of the bladder, after the battle of Monterey. One of the patients died on the sixteenth, one on the twenty-second, and one on the twenty-third day.

There are, however, upon record, a considerable number of recoveries after similar accidents; sufficient, at least, to encourage a hope even in the most unpromising case.

CHAPTER X.

AMPUTATIONS.

THERE are several questions relating to amputations, which need to be considered briefly, and in their proper order.

First.—*What conditions of the limb in army practice demand amputation?*

Simple fracture of a limb, it is unnecessary to say, does not demand amputation.

A fracture complicated with considerable laceration of the skin, or of the skin and muscular tissue, does not of necessity demand amputation.

A fracture, with laceration of the main arterial trunk supplying the limb, does not necessarily demand amputation. If the artery can be tied, the limb may be saved, and the fracture treated successfully.

A fracture, accompanied with the laceration of one or more of the principal nervous trunks, does not always demand amputation, yet it is a graver accident than the one last supposed.

A fracture, complicated with a destruction of both the principal arterial and nervous trunks, occurring in the course of a large limb, like the thigh, the leg, the arm, or the forearm, renders amputation necessary.

Similar lesions, without a fracture, render amputation almost equally imperative.

Comminuted fractures, accompanied with extensive

lesions of the soft parts, or with a rupture of either the principal artery or the principal nerves, in the case of large limbs, generally demand amputation in army practice.

Compound fractures, with either of the above complications, in large limbs, generally demand amputation.

Compound fractures of the *femur*, without other complications, in army practice, *generally* demand amputation.

Fractures accompanied with extensive and violent contusion, demand amputation oftener than the same fractures accompanied with open laceration.

In army practice, gunshot wounds which penetrate the shoulder-joint, the elbow-joint, or the wrist-joint, demand either amputation or resection. (Guthrie says, that an arm will endure almost any amount of injury, without demanding amputation.)

Gunshot wounds penetrating the hip-joint are generally fatal, yet amputation may be practised under some very favorable circumstances. Resection also presents a feeble ground for hope.

Gunshot wounds of the knee or ankle-joint demand either amputation or resection. The knee more certainly than the ankle; and amputation is more often required than resection. Guthrie has seen no recovery from a gunshot wound of the knee-joint, unless the limb was amputated. Nearly all army surgeons confirm this experience.

Gunshot wounds, in which the ball does not actually enter the joint, but in which the bone is struck above or below, and the line of fracture extends into the joint, are subject to nearly the same rules as that class of cases in which the ball enters the joint; but the rule is less imperative.

Gunshot wounds penetrating the carpal bones do not generally exact amputation; but the same wounds penetrating the tarsal bones, generally render amputation necessary.

Gunshot wounds through or between the phalanges of the fingers or toes, or through the bones themselves, are often cured without amputation. Similar wounds of the fingers or toes do not in general result so favorably; but the rule in this latter case cannot be stated very positively.

Second.—*The point at which the amputation is to be made.*

This must depend mostly upon the part of the limb which has suffered injury; but in general we may say, at as low a point as will be safe; or in other words, we would state the rule to be, to *save as much of the limb as possible.* Yet in no case should the life be put at hazard for the sake of a limb, much less for a small portion of a limb.

There are two reasons why we adopt the rule above stated. *First*, because the longer the stump, the more useful it will be to the possessor; and *Second*, because experience has shown that the nearer an amputation is made to the trunk and the larger the circumference of the limb, the greater is the danger to life. Thus, according to Malgaigne, only one death occurred from twenty-six amputations of one of the smaller toes; seven deaths from forty-six amputations of the great toe; nine from thirty-eight partial amputations of the foot; one hundred and six from one hundred and ninety-two amputations of the leg, and one hundred and twenty-six from two hundred and one amputations of the thigh. Again, in the Crimea the mortality after amputations of the thigh, in a certain number of cases, was as follows: Lower third, fifty-six per cent.; middle third, sixty per cent.; upper third, eighty-six per cent.; hip, one hundred per cent. (twenty-three cases*). The same law of relative mortality was

* Stephen Smith, Surgeon to the Bellevue Hospital, and Professor of the Principles of Surgery, in a paper on hip-joint amputations, has brought

observed by the British surgeons in amputations of the upper extremities. After amputation of the forearm, seven per cent. died; of the upper arm, nineteen; and of the shoulder-joint, thirty-five per cent.

The mortality after amputation of the femur through the upper third, is stated to be eighty-six per cent., but it is quite probable that it was much higher. McLeod says that he never saw himself any case recover in which the amputation was beyond doubt in the upper third. The French and Russians also found these amputations so hopeless that they almost abandoned them.

In certain instances, however, we find it convenient or necessary to deviate from the rule which we have established to "save as much of the limb as possible."

There is no reason to suppose that disarticulations, or amputations made through joints, are any more dangerous than amputations made by section of the bone; and on the field, time is of so much consequence, that we can well afford to sacrifice a small portion of a phalanx, by disarticulation at the nearest sound joint, rather than make the delay necessary for the application of the saw. Nor is it scarcely worth while to attempt to save a few of the carpal bones, when the disarticulation can be effected at the wrist-joint so much more speedily and neatly; indeed, if they were saved, they would, under any circumstances, add little or nothing to the value of the limb.

Other things being equal, we might prefer to amputate just below the elbow-joint, rather than through the joint, in order to save an inch or two of the radius and ulna; but the dangers to the patient are not, we think, precisely equal.

together ninety-eight cases, of which fifty-six proved fatal; a ration of mortality of only fifty-seven and a half per cent. (*N. Y. Jour. Med.*, Sept. 1852.) In the Mexican campaign all amputations at the hip-joint terminated fatally.

It is safer to amputate through the joint, than at a point in such close proximity below, since by the latter method we expose the patient to the danger of inflammation extending from the wound upwards into the unopened, but more or less disturbed articulation. The same remarks apply to amputations made an inch or two below the head of the humerus. It will be better, generally, to disarticulate at the shoulder-joint. This latter operation was made in the Crimea, from the 1st of April to the end of the war, one hundred and two times, and it was followed by death in only twenty-five cases.

We would, upon the field or in civil practice, amputate toes only at the articulations; occasionally we may make an exception in favor of the first phalanx of the great toe, which can with advantage sometimes be divided through its middle portion.

In amputating at the foot we may remove all the metatarsal bones, according to the method recommended by Heys; or we may separate the tarsal bones between the calcaneum and astragalus on the one hand, and the cuboides and scaphoides on the other, as practised by Chopart; a portion only of the calcaneum may be saved, as in the operation of Pirogoff, or the complete disarticulation may be effected at the ankle-joint, as improved and recommended by Syme.

If, however, it becomes a question of amputation within one inch above the joint, or six or eight inches, we would unhesitatingly declare in favor of the latter, since the stump is not so likely to ulcerate, or to leave a tender cicatrix, exfoliation of the bone is not so apt to occur, and the power of the leg as a lever is not materially diminished. Indeed, we ought to say that upon the field we would prefer this point to disarticulation according to the method of Syme, since the latter exacts on the part of the operator the utmost care, and requires, for its skilful performance, a good deal of time; besides this, experience has shown that Syme's operation does better when it is made for chronic disease of the foot, than when made for traumatic lesions. Pirogoff's modification of Syme's operation is liable to the same criticism.

We would not amputate within an inch of the knee-joint, for the same reason that has been given for preferring not to amputate just below the elbow-joint. It has been found to be extra-hazardous.

Amputation through the knee-joint is not objectionable, provided a small portion of the lower end of the femur is at the same time sawed off, as has been recommended by Mr. Syme. This affords a more even stump, and does not increase the danger. Baudens says that his experience in the Crimea enables him to affirm that disarticulation of the knee ought always to be preferred to amputation of the thigh. When this operation is made, the patella should be preserved, and great care must be taken that the flaps are ample, so as to cover in completely the expanded surface of bone. Of eighty-six cases brought together, in the Nov. No. 1852, of the *N. Y. Jour. Med.*, by Prof. Stephen Smith, forty-nine resulted in recovery, and thirty-seven died, giving forty-three per cent. as the ratio of mortality.

Amputations ought to be made through the trochanters of the femur rather than through the hip-joint. We have seen that all of the cases of this latter operation, twenty-three in number, made by the British and French surgeons in the Crimea, proved fatal. Yet it is not certain but that it would be better in all cases of gunshot wounds occurring in the upper third of the thigh, to adopt it as a rule not to amputate; so little encouragement do the statistics of these amputations, made by army surgeons, afford.

Amputations made through the cancellous structures, near the ends of long bones, are less dangerous than those made through the shafts. This is explained by the fact that amputations through the tubular portions of the bone expose to diffuse inflammation and suppuration of the medullary canal and consequent pyemia.

Third.—*The method of amputation.*

Upon this point surgeons remain greatly divided. Velpeau, Guthrie, Tavernier, Sir Astley Cooper, Ben. Bell, Charles Bell, Gibson of Philadelphia, Paul F. Eve of Tennessee, and many other distinguished surgeons at home and abroad, prefer the circular method. In France this mode is generally practised.

Liston, Lizars, Fergusson, and Syme, who may be said to represent the Edinburgh school, prefer the flap method. In this country it is very generally adopted, especially by the younger class of surgeons.

Without entering into a discussion of the relative advantages of these two methods in *general* practice, or attempting to reconcile the conflicting opinions of the two parties, we shall content ourselves by affirming our belief that both methods have their special applications; and that, in general, the choice may be safely left to the judgment of any intelligent surgeon.

In relation to their application to *military* practice, however, it seems necessary to make one or two special explanations.

In nearly all amputations made upon the field, where haste is demanded, the flap amputations have greatly the advantage. They can be made in much less time, and where time is a consideration of the greatest moment, they are greatly to be preferred.

If, however, time is of less importance, as it will be whenever the number of surgeons is properly proportioned to the number of the wounded, and the patient is to be transported immediately or soon after the operation a long distance, the preference ought to be given to the circular amputation, at least in the case of all larger limbs.

The heavy flaps attached to the end of the limb, disturbed by incessant motion, loosen, and become gangrenous or ulcerate. This was the experience of the Crimean surgeons, where soldiers were transported long distances by land after amputation; and even when carried upon transports to Scutari, the same fact was observed.

Fourth.—*The period of time at which the amputation ought to be made.*

The "shock" is that condition of the nervous system which immediately ensues upon certain injuries in certain persons, characterized by coldness of the surface, pallor, tremors, a wild, anxious expression of the face, small, irregular, and feeble pulse, sighing respiration, partial or complete paralysis of the bladder and sometimes of other organs, mental disquiet or apprehension, incoherent speech, etc.; which condition may continue a longer or shorter period, but usually, unless severe, disappears in a few hours. When the accident is of a more grave character, no reaction occurs, and the patient dies immediately, or within a short time. In general it may be said, that if reaction does not occur within twenty-four or at most forty-eight hours, the patient will die.

In some cases the occurrence of the shock seems to be delayed, the depressing influence of the injury not being felt until some little time after. Such, at least, is the opinion of Mr. McLeod, who affirms that he knows of several well authenticated cases which prove the correctness of this position. For ourselves, we confess that we have never met with these examples, except where some visceral lesion or the rupture of a large blood-vessel has accompanied the accident. It is true that men often faint after a few minutes, or after removal, and when they have had time to contemplate their situation, who seemed undisturbed at first; and in other cases a severe and prolonged irritation from a spicula of bone has steadily aggravated the signs of depression and of shock; but we think these cannot with propriety be termed examples of delayed shock. We do not intend, however, to deny that the nervous agitations may be delayed in some cases, but only to express our conviction that the condition to which our attention has been called by these gentlemen is a rare phenomenon.

Surgeons who hold to the frequent occurrence of delayed shock, recognise in this an argument in favor of *immediate* amputation, in a great majority of cases; and certainly, assuming the premises to be correct, the argument seems not unsound. Says McLeod, "if this precious moment could be seized at all times, and that operation performed under chloroform, which assists so much in warding off the 'ebranlement' we fear, how much more successful would our results prove, than under other circumstances they can ever be."

The idea of immediate amputation did not, however, originate with those who maintain that the shock may be, and is, in fact, often delayed. Ambrose Paré urged that amputation should be made while the wounded were in sight of the battle-field; and Richard Wiseman, Sergeant Surgeon to Charles the Second, says, "if you decide to operate, do so at once, while the soldier is in heat and in mettle."

Larrey, indeed, seemed to regard amputation as the proper remedy for this peculiar condition of the nervous system. "I have lost," said he, "a great number of soldiers, because, although operated upon within the first twenty-four hours, yet the operations had been made too late. * * * It is then demonstrated that the commotion, far from being a contra-indication to primitive amputation, ought to decide the surgeon in its favor. * * * The effects of the commotion, far from being aggravated, diminish and disappear insensibly after the operation."

Dubor, who served in America during the War of the Revolution, states, that "American surgeons amputated at once, and lost but few, but that the French delayed and lost many."

In regard to this question, it is our opinion, also, that amputations may be made in some cases immediately, or as soon as possible after the receipt of the injury; as, for example, when a limb is nearly torn off, and a dangerous hæmorrhage, which cannot be arrested, is occurring; or when spiculæ of bone, such as neither the forceps nor fingers can extricate, are causing intense suffering. In all cases of injuries to small limbs, such as the fingers and toes, immediate amputation is proper; and in a considerable number of cases of injuries to larger limbs, when it is clearly seen that the patient is not faint, or depressed, or suffering under great nervous agitation. But we cannot accept of the doctrines of Paré, Wiseman, Larrey, McLeod, and others, without liberal qualifications, and a careful specification of the cases to which their rules are to be made applicable.

It may be that, as Hutcheson declares, the condition which we term shock, is not so frequently present as has been generally supposed, even after severe injuries; or that, as McLeod maintains, there is generally an interval, longer or shorter, between the receipt of the injury and the accession of the nervous commotion. These points may be safely left open for future inquiry; but upon one thing we must insist, namely, that when the nervous agitation and depression are actually present in any considerable degree, amputation is generally a most dangerous resource. Amputation may then be necessary for the reasons which we have stated, and perhaps for other reasons which we have not noticed, but the necessity is greatly to be deprecated.

Our own experience has been, after at least twenty years of observation in hospital practice, including almost every variety of accidents and of amputations, that amputations of large limbs, made after severe injuries and before reaction has fairly been established, have resulted speedily in the death of the patients.

The cases in which the nervous commotion is "diminished" by an operation, with all deference to the opinion of the distinguished Larrey, we must explain to be those in which the broken bones, fragments of shell, splinters, clothing, or some other foreign substance lying in the track of the wound, are causing pain and perpetuating the irritation. Sometimes, perhaps, it may be the condition of the nerves themselves, or of the other tissues which have suffered laceration, and the clean removal of which by the knife may occasion relief; but such cases would be recognised by the presence of great pain and extraordinary sensibility in the parts, which must lead us at once and naturally to regard amputation as the proper remedy.

In these opinions we think also we are sustained by the observation of a large majority of all practical surgeons, whether in or out of the army.

Our first duty, then, to many who have fallen upon the

field, and who cannot escape amputation, is to comfort and sustain them by words of encouragement, and by the administration of water, wine, brandy, or food; and having dressed the wounds temporarily, to wait patiently the establishment of complete reaction before proceeding to the operation.

As to the value of some delay in certain cases, nothing could be more pertinent than the following communication, which the author has lately received in reply to certain inquiries, from Usher Parsons, of Providence, R. I., surgeon in the United States Navy during the war of 1812. Portions of the letter do not relate especially to the subject of amputation; but it is all of sufficient interest to require of us no apology for its introduction, unabridged, at this place:

"DEAR SIR:—In the battle of Lake Erie, on the 10th of September, 1813, nearly a hundred were wounded; sixty-one of them on board the Lawrence, twenty-three on board the Niagara, and about a dozen in the smaller vessels. There were eleven cases of compound fracture, besides simple fractures, many gunshot wounds, and extensive lacerations, and among them all, several amputations were required. Those wounded on board the Lawrence, were ranged on the upper deck, in the spaces usually occupied by cannon and gun-carriages, which were removed from both sides of the deck, to afford room for mattresses. The only shelter over the wounded thus lodged, was an awning that served to screen them from the sun, and tarpaulins and canvas to spread over and shelter them when it rained.

"To the wounded of the Lawrence were added, after two days, those of the Niagara and of the other small vessels. The whole number of patients requiring a recumbent posture on the deck was about fifty. They remained in the ship fourteen days after the action, and were then landed at Erie, and lodged in a large unfinished court-house, and remained there until cured. Of this ninety-six wounded, only three died, and these were cases of so severe a nature that a surgical operation was not deemed justifiable, and they were left to linger out a few days of miserable existence. This entire success I have ever felt warranted in ascribing to the purity of the air, more than to any other cause.

"Another cause of success worthy of special notice was, the delay of amputations and all severe surgical operations until the system was entirely recovered from the shock of the injury.

"Having sole charge of the wounded of the whole fleet, the other two medical officers being ill, and the wounded being passed down to me faster than I could attend to them in a proper manner, I aimed only to save life during the action, by tying arteries or applying tourniquets to prevent fatal hæmorrhage, and sometimes applying splints as a temporary support to shattered limbs, and in two or three instances small portions of flesh were divided which held a dangling limb, to the great annoyance of the patient. In this state the patients remained until the following morning, under the free use of cordials and anodynes. At sunrise I commenced amputations, and in the course of the whole day and evening was able to finish all operations and dressings, and I believe do justice to each. On the following day I visited the other vessels, and brought all their wounded on board the Lawrence, and treated them in like manner. Now, as all but the three hopeless cases recovered, it was proved beyond a doubt, that the delay of amputations and other severe operations for one, and some even two days, had no unfavorable effect upon the chances of recovery, and probably some lives were saved by it, which would have been lost, had the operations taken place on the day of the injury. I am, however, advancing no new doctrine in this matter, but only adding new facts strikingly illustrative and confirmative of the correctness of those generally received at this day.

"A third cause of success in this action was, the plentiful supply of fresh provisions and vegetables, brought to the fleet from the shores of the Ohio, and of a generous supply of wine and cordials.

"Fourthly. There can be no doubt that cheerful and buoyant spirits, occasioned by victory, contributed not a little to recovery.

"In two other actions I saw much to confirm the foregoing opinions. In an attack on Mackinac the following year by Col. Croghran's small army, transported thither in our vessels, the number wounded was less than that on Lake Erie. Our vessels were crowded and afforded no suitable lodgings for the patients—the air became foul—diet was salt meat and dry biscuit, with no fresh vegetables, and added to this, was the failure of our enterprise, we being repulsed. Consequently the wounds acted unkindly, and some died, that under favorable circumstances might have been saved.

"In a third action opposite Black Rock near Buffalo, nearly a hundred of our sailors crossed the Niagara in a cold November night to take a battery by storm, preparatory to the crossing of General Smyth's army to take Upper Canada. The sailors succeeded, with the loss of seven killed and about thirty wounded. The distance is about one mile across the river, and the wounded were much chilled in recrossing in open boats. The apartments for receiving them were very small and ill ventilated, but this was slightly remedied by a wood fire, which served to establish a current of fresh air from without. There were extensive suppurations, and some deaths of persons who, in favorable circumstances, might have recovered.

"You inquire the result of my experience in amputation for *tetanus*. I think unfavorably of it. I have amputated twice without any benefit. The disease has extended to the spinal cord. Actual cautery over this with an iron brought to a white heat is reported to have saved life in some cases, but I have seen no case of a cure, by any treatment, of an established *tetanus*. For prevention of traumatic tetanus after a battle, I deem it of great importance to graduate the covering and clothing of the wounded, according to the temperature of the air. Hot days succeeded by cold nights are among the prominent causes of tetanus in armies and in ships of war.

"Yours very respectfully,

"USHER PARSONS."

Primary amputations, in the meaning of the term as now employed by most surgeons, are amputations made during the first twelve, twenty-four, or forty-eight hours, but not until after the severity of the shock has passed off, and more or less complete reaction has taken place in the general system. When writers speak of "primary" amputations, therefore, they intend generally to exclude from consideration "immediate" amputations.

Secondary amputations, as distinguished from primary, are those made, not immediately or soon after complete reaction has ensued, but after the inflammation consequent upon the injury has subsided, when perhaps suppuration has already commenced, or even at a later day.

The next question to be determined, then, is as to the relative safety of amputations made after reaction has ensued, and prior to the occurrence of inflammation, on the one hand, and amputations made after the inflammation has subsided, on the other hand.

In *civil* practice, secondary amputations are almost universally admitted to have been more successful than primary, the only real point at issue being, what has been the result of experience upon this point in *army* and *naval* practice; and we shall presently see that here surgeons differ pretty widely, but that at the present moment the great weight of authority preponderates upon the side of primary amputations. In fact, if we would look for advocates of secondary amputations in military practice, we shall have to seek for them mainly among army surgeons of the last, or in the early part of the present century. Faure, who was at the battle of Fontenoy, says, "Amputate after the subsidence of the first symptoms, and when suppuration is produced." John Hunter adopted the same views. Baron Percy, in 1792, taught a similar doctrine; and in our own century, Blandin and Mann have arrayed themselves upon the same side: while Petit, Le Dran, Bromfield, Boucher, Guthrie, Hennen, Roux, Rush, Armand, and a host of others, have decided in favor of primary amputations.

Dr. John L. Stone, surgeon to the Bellevue Hospital, New York, in the November No. for 1849 of the *New York Journal of Medicine*, has given the most complete statistical record of the results of primary and secondary amputations which we have seen; and he sums up his conclusions, in part, as follows:

Primary amputations of the upper extremities are to be preferred both in military and civil practice, being more successful than secondary in both.

Primary amputations of the lower extremities are twice as successful as secondary in military practice.

There is another view of this important question which needs to be stated, and for the presentation of which, in a reliable and statistical form, we are also indebted to Dr. Stone. We refer to a comparison of the results of both primary and secondary amputations, with no amputations at all!

We believe that, after Bilquer, Malgaigne was the first to make the startling announcement that in the attempt to save the limbs, we run no greater risk than we do in amputating them; his opinions being founded upon his experience in the campaign in Poland, "where, in an army of

80,000 men, neither he nor his colleagues succeeded in saving a case after amputation of the lower extremities;" and also upon certain results furnished by the statistics of the Parisian hospitals, where, during a period of three years, the mortality was seventy-five per cent.

It is well known that after the "Astor House Riot" in the city of New York, all of those whose limbs were amputated died. The amputations were primary. While, according to the statements published by Dr. George D. Gibb, of the wounded in the Parisian hospitals after the revolution of June, 1848, only six deaths occurred in compound fractures of the thigh out of the twelve cases in which an attempt was made to save the limb. These were all gunshot wounds; but it must not be forgotten that so far as the management of the patients was concerned, subsequent to their injuries, they were in the conditions of civil practice.

M. Baudens, surgeon of Val de Grace, and late Army Surgeon in Algiers, and Drs. Walker and Pierson, of Massachusetts, have also done much towards arresting the indiscriminate sacrifice of limbs after complicated fractures. We are not, however, at present prepared to decide all the points in this delicate question, especially as applied to Army Surgery; and while we may hope that the facts brought together with so much care by Dr. Stone may save some limbs, and perhaps lives, by judicious treatment, and without resort to amputation, we may be permitted to express a hope, also, that it will not lead surgeons to indecision and fatal delays, especially upon the field. Certainly we are in no danger of adopting the extreme views of Bilquer and Malgaigne, by rejecting amputations altogether.

In army practice, just here is one of the great points of difference as compared with civil practice; in the former, patients have to be moved often, and to great distances, which render quiet to the limb, and many other hygienic attentions, actually impossible; yet it is upon these alone that the surgeon can rely to save mutilated members. Moreover, it is a matter of great importance for the safety of other patients crowded into the same wards, that suppuration and animal decomposition shall be prevented as far as this can be done. A military ward, filled with suppurating and sloughing wounds, would soon become untenantable by the generation of poisonous gases. In these circumstances, almost peculiar to military practice, we see some good reasons why primary amputations are likely to prove more successful, and why army surgeons have so generally conceded to them the preference.

If an attempt is made to save a limb badly lacerated and broken, certain conditions in the treatment are necessary to success.

All projecting pieces of bone which cannot be easily replaced and are not firmly attached to the soft parts, must be at once cut or sawn away.

All foreign substances, such as fragments of balls or other missiles, pieces of cloth, wadding, dirt, &c., must be removed.

Any portions of integument, fascia, or muscles, which are entangled in the wound, and prevent a thorough exploration, or may obstruct the free escape of blood or of matter, must be freely divided.

Counter-openings must be made at once, or at an early period after the formation of matter, to permit its easy escape.

The limb must be placed in an easy position, and not confined by tight bandages, or forcibly extended by apparatus.

Inflammation must be prevented or controlled by constitutional and local means, and especially by the use of water lotions whenever its employment is practicable.

If joints are implicated, they must be laid freely open, and placed at perfect rest, without adhesive straps, bandages, or other means of compression.

CHAPTER XI.

ON THE EMPLOYMENT OF ANÆSTHETICS IN AMPUTATIONS AND OTHER SURGICAL OPERATIONS, AFTER GUNSHOT INJURIES.

McLeod, as we have already noticed, maintains that anæsthetics do not generally increase the shock, or the nervous depression consequent upon severe injuries. He has reaffirmed his confidence in these agents, and especially in chloroform, by the following unequivocal language: "If we believe, as I certainly do, that by the use of this anæsthetic, all fear of intensifying the shock is obviated," &c.; and Baudens assures us that "they had no fatal accidents to deplore from its use, although during the Eastern campaign chloroform was employed thirty thousand times or more."

Such testimony demands respectful attention, and cannot be rejected except upon the most satisfactory evidence of its fallacy or unsoundness. We believe that in the main it must be accepted as it stands, but there are points in the testimony which need explanation, and certain facts of experience which will in some degree weaken its authority.

M. Baudens has no doubt said honestly that so far as he has been informed or has himself seen, no fatal cases have occurred from the use of chloroform in the Crimea; and yet, judging from the number of deaths from this cause already reported in civil practice, it is fair to assume that some fatal cases have occurred, also, in the Crimea. What means of information does M. Baudens possess, which can be considered reliable, as to the number of deaths which it may have occasioned in the trenches, where it was constantly given by inexperienced assistants, and who might not always be able to distinguish between the effects of the injury and of the chloroform?

Admitting, however, that in no case did death result immediately from its use, there is another question to be determined to which these writers do not allude, and which we think has heretofore been kept too much out of sight by those who have spoken upon the subject of anæsthesia in general—we refer to the question whether its after effects upon the system and upon the wounds are favorable or unfavorable.

Says McLeod: "I never saw one case among our most numerous amputations in which primary adhesion took place throughout the whole surface of the flaps." Is not this a most unparalleled experience? Do the annals of surgery furnish another such example? Why did these wounds so uniformly refuse to unite by first intention? It is in vain to invoke by way of explanation, bad diet, fatigue, exposure, discontent, cold, heat, moisture, ill-ventilated hospitals, or crowded transports; these were all, at one time or another, active agents in the production of disease in the Crimea, but none of them were constantly present; and especially during the last year of the campaign, thanks to the intelligence of the English medical officers, and to the energy of the British nation—were nearly all of these depressing influences absent. "Every man was then in health and vigor—literally full of lusty life—and actually rejoicing in his strength."

We submit, therefore, whether it is not proper to look for some other more constant cause for such remarkable results, than any or all of those which have been enumerated—a cause which might be found acting, perhaps, solely upon the wounded soldiers. Before these injuries were received they were all "full of lusty life," but, immediately that a surgical operation was made, the functions of life were so much lowered that the natural processes of repair were uniformly interrupted or completely arrested.

It is very natural, while contemplating the virtues of one of the most valuable discoveries ever made in medicine, that we should overlook and be reluctant to admit its defects. The danger is indeed very great that we shall do so; and in the name of humanity, we demand for this question a most careful consideration.

We ought, perhaps, to mention that in one Division of the British army, chloroform was not so much used as in the others, "from an aversion to it entertained by the principal medical officer of the Division—a gentleman of very extensive experience."

We have many times had occasion to notice the appearance presented by the stump immediately after an amputation made upon a patient completely narcotised by chloroform. The muscles hang out much as they do in operations made upon the cadaver; they never quiver nor retract, nor, in some cases, is the retraction of the muscles completely accomplished until after several hours or even days. Can this condition of the wound be favorable to early union of the surfaces? It bleeds freely under these circumstances, but it is seldom we shall find any lymph deposited upon the surface, even when it has been allowed to remain open an hour or more. We have noticed, also, the prostrated condition of the patient, consequent plainly upon the action of the anæsthetic, and continuing several hours or days; and we think we are not mistaken in supposing that of late, since the introduction of anæsthetics, we have seen fewer examples of union by first intention, and more of suppuration, with also purulent infection, or pyæmia.

The following remarks on the employment of anæsthetics in military surgery, are from the pen of Dr. Z. Pitcher, Surgeon in the United States Army, during the war of 1812, and at present the surgeon to St. Mary's Hospital, Detroit; they constitute a portion of a private communication made to the author a few days since. They correspond so nearly with our own views that we shall take the liberty of quoting them entire:

"You will observe, that in what I have said on this subject, I have spoken only in such general terms as will serve to convey my idea of the principle by which my own conduct has been governed, and by which I would direct the action of others, and that I have not affected the precision of a clinical instructor. Such cases as I can most distinctly recall, illustrative of what I have already said, I propose to speak of in connexion with the use of anæsthetics in cases of shock, the effects of which I think it my duty to place on record, they being the results of my own experience in its administration, where the subject was approaching the state of collapse.

"Whenever there is sufficient force in the circulation, and nervous activity enough to sustain the patient, I would give my voice with the general judgment of the medical profession, by which the use of anæsthetics in the severer operations of surgery is sustained. But regarding them as poisons of a sedative class, which, when introduced in the blood, produce cerebral exhaustion and cardiac syncope, if they do not change the physical and vital properties of the blood itself, I feel obliged, in discharging a duty incident to a compliance with your request, to remonstrate against their use in cases of syncope, or nervous exhaustion.

"Two men were conveyed to the hospital under circumstances so nearly identical, that I could scarcely say wherein they differed, unless in temperament, each having had a leg carried away so near the knee that amputation was performed above the joint. They were nearly of the same age, they had good constitutions, and neither of them was intemperate. One was put under the influence of chloroform, and the other not. Neither made favorable progress, but the one subjected to the influence of the anæsthetic came out of that condition with increased prostration, and never regained what he had thus lost. The other rallied slowly, and union of the wound took place very late. The increased prostration in the first case may be explained on either of two hypotheses; but the latter example, strengthened by others, inclines me to impute the increased prostration to the anæsthetic, rather than to the operation.

"The case of a seaman who was brought into St. Mary's Hospital, furnishes so good an instance of the inapplicability of anæsthetics in some of the severest injuries, and affords so striking an example of the ability of a vigorous constitution to emerge from the most desperate condition, that I am tempted to mention it, although it belongs to maritime, rather than to military surgery. ——— was standing on the deck of a propeller directly over the boiler at the time of its explosion. The uplifting force caused a compound dislocation of the knee, the condyles of the femur being thrust forward, tearing up the ligamentum patellæ, the capsular and crucial ligaments. The leg and thigh were held together by the tendons constituting the outer and the inner hamstrings, and the vessels and nerves lying in the popliteal space. He had a severe scalp wound also, and with it signs of concussion of the brain. The cerebral symptoms blending with the general phenomena of shock rendered the use of chloroform entirely inadmissible, and the jactitation of the patient made it equally necessary to remove the leg. A very good reaction followed the operation, the stump healed kindly, and the man seemed to be rapidly recovering, when symptoms of cerebral suppuration supervened, and put an end to his existence."

Dr. J. B. Porter, Surgeon U. S. Army, in a communication to the *Amer. Jour. Med. Sci.*, 1852, states, that after a fair trial at the General Hospital, Vera Cruz, in 1847, anæsthetics were entirely given up; and he adds—

"It may be well questioned whether anæsthetics are not calculated to produce injurious effects in all important amputations; but they certainly do so in operations performed for gunshot wounds. M. Velpeau says: 'Chloroform evidently depresses the nervous system, and as great prostration always exists in patients who have received gunshot wounds, it is advisable to refrain from any anæsthetic means.' Mr. Alcock refers to the cases of soldiers wounded in battle, where the excitement is such as to carry them through almost any operation. I regret that Mr. Alcock's paper is not before me. These are the cases spoken of by Mr. Guthrie: 'Soldiers in general are anxious to undergo an operation when they find it inevitable, and frequently press it before the proper time; that is, before they have sufficiently recovered the shock of the injury.' These are the cases which require a little more time, some 'encouraging words,' and perhaps a little wine, or brandy and water; but no anæsthetics, for the patients are already sufficiently depressed.

"There are two sets of cases; in one (Velpeau's), the shock to the nervous system is great, from which the patient may not recover, and the use of anæsthetics would be awfully destructive; in the other class, they are unnecessary, and would prove useless and injurious. In the flap operation they must prove more injurious than in the circular; from the fact that muscle forms almost the entire covering for the stump; and the contractility of the muscular tissue is for a time almost annihilated, to be recovered irregularly at irregular intervals. Further, after the use of these agents, wounds do not heal so readily by the first intention.

"M. Jobert, on the use of ether, states that the local inflammation has proved less, and that union by the first intention has been prevented. I am able to bear testimony to the correctness of M. Jobert's statement.

"I must be permitted to refer to the *Transactions of the American Medical Association* for 1851, pp. 271, 272, 315, 323. In the Massachusetts General Hospital :—

"'It does not appear that the fatal results of amputation have at all diminished by the introduction of anæsthetic agents.'

"New York Hospital :—

"'The general mortality has been for three years and a quarter forty per centum. As regards the method of operating, we observe that the amputations of the thigh, in which the fatality was as high as thirteen in seventeen, were all flap operations. Eleven of the leg were removed by the circular, one died; while of four by the flap, two died.'

"That is, nine per cent. in one set of cases, and fifty per cent. in the other.

"'In almost every case chloroform or ether was employed; but, while it is admitted that anæsthetics may have had some influence in the increased mortality in the New York Hospital over preceding years, since union by the first intention was now much less frequently observed; still it is to be remembered that hospital gangrene, entirely unknown before, and purulent cachexia and erysipelas, extensively prevailed there during the past three years.'

"Could the anæsthetics have had an influence in producing the 'hospital gangrene, entirely unknown before,' and the 'purulent cachexia and erysipelas,' as well as prevent union by the first intention?

"Dr. Lente, Resident Surgeon of the New York Hospital, says:—'In almost every case, however, either chloroform or ether was employed; generally the former, until the occurrence of a fatal case from it in this hospital; afterwards the latter, from which we have never had any bad consequences, and which has never failed to prove effectual. * * * Anæsthetics came into general use about the period of the commencement of these statistics. May not the employment of these have had its influence upon the mortality? This is a very important question. We do not deny that it may have had some influence in augmenting the fatality of operations; but we have seen no reason to infer that it has, except perhaps the fact that union by adhesion seems to have been much less frequent since the introduction of anæsthetics into this hospital than before. Whether the two are in the relation of cause and effect, it is, we fear, impossible to determine at present.'

"In an unhealthy atmosphere or climate, the healing of wounds by adhesive union is doubly important, for obvious reasons; and I have often regretted that etherization was so much resorted to in capital operations at Vera Cruz during a portion of 1847; nor can I avoid congratulating both the patients and myself, that, before the summer had passed away, its employment was wholly abandoned. Anæsthetics poison the blood and depress the nervous system; and, in consequence, hæmorrhage is much more apt to occur, and union by adhesion is prevented."

Finally, after comparing our own experience with that of others, we will state our belief and conclusions as follows:—Anæsthetics are of inestimable value in their efforts as remedial agents, and in their power to extinguish sensibility, temporarily, and especially during the performance of severe surgical operations; but we prefer ether to chloroform, as being the least liable to destroy life; and we would never employ either when the system was greatly prostrated by disease, or by the shock of a recent injury, unless the patient exhibited an unconquerable dread of the pain of the operation, or the operation was likely to prove exceedingly painful.

It is our opinion, also, that anæsthetics sometimes, and especially chloroform, prevent the union of wounds by adhesion, or by "first intention."

CHAPTER XII.

HOSPITAL GANGRENE.

(*Syn.* Hospital Sore. Phagedæna Gangrenosa. Pourriture d'hôpital. La gangrene humide des hôpitaux. Putrid, contagious, malignant, gangrenous ulcer.)

Causes.—The causes of hospital gangrene are, overcrowding of patients in confined and filthy apartments, the congregating of men in ill-ventilated barracks, encamping vast multitudes in too narrow limits, and where the winds do not have free access to all the tents, bad or innutritious food, stimulating drinks, great loss of blood, the shock of a severe injury, a scorbutic state of the system, insufficient attention to cleanliness and to the dressing of wounds, mental depression, acrid and irritating applications, motion or mechanical irritation, a hot and moist climate, exposure to a cold and damp atmosphere, specific contagion.

There is no evidence that it is ever due to a general epidemic condition of the atmosphere, but it may originate from poisons generated in foul wards, and which pervade the atmosphere of these apartments, after which it has the power of propagation by infection or inoculation. It may be conveyed from one person to another by the sponge, or by pieces of cloth used in dressing the wounds; and its infectious character is so active that when once it has made its appearance in an apartment, nothing but the complete removal of the affected, followed by the most thorough and searching cleansing and ventilation, will suffice for its arrest, or prevent its reappearance whenever the rooms are again occupied.

Signs.—When the hospital gangrene attacks an unbroken surface, it commences as a vesicle, filled with bloody ichor, small, and of a dark color, attended with a hot, stinging pain; this breaks, leaving a circular ulceration, with sharp edges. The ulceration having thus begun, it extends generally with great rapidity, accompanied with sloughing.

When, as is usually the case, it makes its primary invasion upon the open surface or margins of a wound, the part affected assumes a grey or greenish color, becomes soft, swollen, and pultaceous, discharging a thin, yellowish, greenish, or brown, and very offensive matter, or the surface ceases to discharge matter and becomes dry. This suspension of secretion generally precedes the ichorous discharge. The surrounding integuments are thickened with an œdematous swelling, and of a livid or erysipelatous complexion.

The edges of the sore are everted, abrupt, and circular; unless covered with sloughs, which are tenacious, and cannot be removed without violence. The neighboring glands inflame and sometimes suppurate.

The progress of the sloughing and ulceration, when the disease is fully developed, is, in most cases, exceedingly rapid; integuments, muscles, tendons, fascia, and finally the arteries, yielding unresistingly to its ravages. Hennen says, the arteries are most likely to give way about the eleventh day. In the early stages of the malady bleeding seldom occurs.

The constitutional symptoms sometimes precede the local appearance of the malady, but more often follow. In either case they are generally formidable; at first, and in a few examples, the type of the fever is sthenic or inflammatory;

but in a majority of cases it is asthenic from the outset. Whether the fever is sthenic or asthenic at the period of its announcement, as the disease progresses the signs of depression become marked, and the patient rapidly sinks into a typhoid condition.

Treatment.—The preventive treatment consists in the avoidance of all those general or specific causes which we have seen occasion the malady. In the Crimean war, hospital gangrene only appeared at Scutari during the first winter, and in a mild form. Its appearance at this time was ascribed to the very filthy and crowded condition of the barrack hospitals. Dispersion and cleanliness soon completely arrested its further progress.

Patients affected with hospital gangrene should be at once removed to remote and isolated wards, or to detached buildings; the affected wards should be ventilated, cleansed, and whitewashed, or thoroughly painted; each patient should have his own sponge, and in no case should the dressings be allowed to be used twice, even after thorough washing. It is better to make it a rule to burn them as soon as they are removed.

When it breaks out in an encampment the tents should be thoroughly cleansed and ventilated, and the straw daily changed; or they should be separated further from each other; and if these means fail, the encampment, if practicable, should be broken up, and changed to some more healthy location.

The curative means are both constitutional and local.

The constitutional measures to be employed must depend upon the character of the constitutional affection, the condition of the patient, and perhaps many other circumstances.

Occasionally, in the first stage, it may be found necessary to bleed; more often cathartics are indicated, mercury is always injurious—but, as a general rule, especially when it is prevailing in an endemic form, tonics, stimulants, and a nutritious diet are demanded from the beginning.

Hennen, Boggic, Baird, Ballingall, and some others, regard bleeding as the most important medicinal agent in the early stages of this malady. Sir James McGregor relies much upon emetics, and Blackadder, who maintains that the affection is almost entirely local in its character, places little reliance upon constitutional means of any kind, but depends chiefly upon topical applications, especially the arsenical solutions.

The local applications which have been found most useful, are concentrated nitric acid, applied freely to the sloughing or ulcerating surface, caustic potass, actual cautery, or some other active escharotic; after which the sore should be dressed with lint dipped in a watery solution of opium, or with opium cerate. A weak solution of the chloride of soda, or of lime, is also sometimes useful. Yeast or charcoal poultices aid much in correcting the intolerable fœtor.

Dead or sloughing portions of flesh may be cut away, but not detached by violence. In no case should amputation be practised during the progress of the malady, or until the general system has sufficiently rallied to endure the shock of such an operation.

CHAPTER XIII.

DYSENTERY.

THE fact that in not a few military campaigns disease has occasioned a vastly greater loss of life than the sword of the enemy, cannot be too forcibly impressed on medical and other army officers. Losses by the sword are under the control of the army surgeon only in so far as he may save life by the skilful and judicious management of the wounded; but destruction from disease is controllable, to a greater or less extent, by proper hygienic management, in conjunction with the successful treatment of the sick. The importance of preventing, as well as curing disease, should be impressed upon other officers as well as upon those of the medical staff, because the co-operation of both is requisite in carrying out efficient measures for protection against disease.

Among the various diseases which past experience has shown to be destructive to troops, the affection which heads this chapter holds a high rank. Dr. Watson, in his lectures on the principles and practice of physic, says of dysentery: "There is no single malady which is so crippling to an army in the field as this. Sir James M'Gregor, to whom was intrusted the superintendence of the medical department of the army on the two greatest services on which the military force of this country has, of late years, been employed, namely, that in Walcheren and that in the Peninsula, calls dysentery the 'scourge of armies,' and 'the most fatal of all' their diseases. In two years and a half the British army in Spain lost no less than 4717 men by this complaint." Loss of life from this disease occurs especially in warm or tropical countries, and more particularly among soldiers accustomed to a northern climate. The fatality from dysentery was very great among our American troops in Mexico in 1847, '8, and '9.

Dysentery occurs as a sporadic and an epidemic disease. In either form it varies exceedingly, as regards gravity, at different times and places. As a sporadic disease, it is rarely fatal in northern climates; but, as an epidemic disease, it is often malignant in all situations, prevailing oftener as an epidemic, and oftener assuming a malignant character in tropical climates. It may be associated with other diseases, especially with the continued and periodical fevers, investing the latter with a fatality which does not intrinsically belong to them. Developed in armies, whether in camp or in the field, in warm latitudes, more particularly during the summer and autumnal seasons, it is apt to prevail extensively as an epidemic, and with extraordinary malignancy. The great fatality in armies, however, is undoubtedly in a measure to be explained by the unpropitious circumstances under which, of necessity, soldiers affected with this disease are treated.

To prevent the development of dysentery, and stay its prevalence when it becomes developed, are among the important objects which claim the attention of the army medical officer. How are these objects to be attained? This question involves another, namely, How far are the causes of dysentery known and controllable? We will consider briefly this latter inquiry.

It may be logically shown that dysentery, at least in its epidemic form, proceeds from a special cause. The inflammatory affection of the mucous membrane of the large intestine does not constitute the disease, but is the definite expression of it. The disease essentially consists in the unknown morbid condition which underlies the local manifestations. The special cause is that which determines this morbid condition. We may logically conclude that the special cause is received from without the body; but of its nature, source, mode of reception, and primary effects within the body, we must confess ignorance. We know, however, as little of most of the external causes of disease. With our present knowledge, we cannot expect to control directly the special cause of dysentery more than other special causes of which we are alike ignorant. But facts go to show that this, like other special causes of disease, often requires for its efficient operation accessory causes; these we can better appreciate, and they are measurably under our control. The practical question, then, is, What are the appreciable accessory causes which predispose to dysentery, or, by operating with the special cause, lead to the development of the disease?

Excessive fatigue or exhaustion predisposes to this as well as to other diseases. The ability to resist the operation of morbific agencies is lessened when the powers of life are prostrated. The exigencies of military service often render this source of predisposition unavoidable; but it is important to spare and support the strength of the soldier as far as practicable. Habits of intemperance and excesses of all kinds predispose in the same way, viz. by diminishing the resistance to the invasion of disease.

Exposure to sudden and great alternations of temperature is a powerful accessory cause. Experience has shown that soldiers are extremely liable to be attacked with dysentery, after lying on the damp ground during the night, having been heated and fatigued by marching or drilling during the day. Much protection against the disease is afforded by obviating dampness from the ground by means of boards, straw, hay, or india-rubber cloth; by a sufficiency of woollen clothing, and by camp fires whenever practicable.

Diet is of great importance. The long-continued and too exclusive use of salted provisions may lead to this disease, as well as to scurvy. These two affections, indeed, may be combined, constituting what has been called scorbutic dysentery. On the other hand, the excessive use of acid or unripe fruits, and of crude or stale vegetables, undoubtedly contributes to the development of the disease. Impure water has been supposed, and reasonably, to contribute to the disease.

Marsh miasmata (so called) render the system susceptible to the special cause of the disease. To such an extent has this fact been apparent, that some have considered dysentery as sometimes attributable directly and exclusively to the miasm which gives rise to periodical fever. It is more rational to regard this in the light of an accessory predisposing cause. It may predispose to dysentery without accumulating in the system sufficiently to occasion intermittent or remittent fever; but dysentery and periodical fever are sometimes presented in combination. As a protection against both forms of disease, care should be taken not to encamp in marshy situations, and, when marching through malarious districts, to select situations as elevated as possible.

Impure air, and especially air contaminated by concentrated emanations from human bodies, may contribute to the development and spread of the disease. The liability to this, as well as other diseases, renders it of great importance in permanent encampments to obviate over-crowding and provide for proper ventilation. This applies, of course, equally to hospitals and to quarters for the well.

The contagiousness of dysentery has been much discussed, and it cannot be considered as fully settled that this disease is never communicable. It may be so under certain circumstances, although in general it is not so. This is true of some other diseases; for example, typhoid fever, which is very rarely transmitted by contagion, and yet is unquestionably thus transmissible. In the present state of uncertainty as regards the possible contagiousness of dysentery, patients should be separated from the well as far as practicable, without giving encouragement to fear of contracting the disease.

Finally, the mental and moral condition of troops is by no means unimportant as regards a predisposition to this in common with other diseases. Buoyancy, hope, confidence, afford, to a certain extent, protection against disease, while the opposite states of the mind favor a predisposition to any morbific agencies to which soldiers are exposed.

Next in importance to preventing the development and prevalence of dysentery, is the appropriate treatment of the disease. To consider this branch of the subject at any length, would not only require too much space, but would be here out of place. Various remedies and methods of treatment have been heretofore advocated. It will suffice to indicate certain points in respect of which the views of practical physicians at the present time differ from those formerly entertained.

Venesection, which was considered as highly important by many up to a recent period, is now resorted to by a very small proportion of practitioners. Local blood-letting by leeches to the abdomen or anus, is sometimes still employed; but, in general, even this measure of depletion is abandoned.

Without proscribing altogether the abstraction of blood, it is not advisable, except in cases which are characterized by high febrile movement, the heart acting with abnormal power, and the patient plethoric or robust. Thus restricted, it will be found applicable to a very few cases only.

Mercury was formerly deemed almost essential in the management of dysentery. It was given with a two-fold object; first, to excite secretion by the liver, and, second, to affect the system. With reference to the former of these objects, the remedy was often given in large doses; and with reference to the latter, it was thought to be important to push its administration to the extent of ptyalism. Some practitioners still employ mercurials, but to less extent than formerly, and by not a few their use has been abandoned.

Of the great number and variety of astringent remedies which have been in use, many are still in vogue. Different practitioners differ as regards the particular articles or preparations to be preferred, and as to the value of this class of remedies.

Cathartics and laxative medicines have always been employed to a greater or less extent. Recently the plan of employing those of the saline class early in the disease, and from time to time during its progress, has been strongly advocated by many practitioners. The objects are to effect a thorough and prompt removal of the contents of the large intestine, and to deplete the portal vascular system directly by means of the liquid evacuations. Clinical experience furnishes abundant evidence of the utility of this plan of treatment; but it should be carefully limited to the objects just stated, and is generally to be resorted to by way of preparation for the administration of opium.

The use of opium in the treatment of dysentery is by no means new, but its efficiency has been better appreciated in this, as well as in other diseases, of late years. The utility of opium, so far as we can understand it, consists in the relief of the pain and tenesmus, and the arrest of the peristaltic movements of the intestines. To secure these objects, proper evacuation of the bowels must be premised, and attended to from time to time during the course of the disease. Experience has shown that in this, as in other diseases, there is a remarkable tolerance of this drug; and that to receive its full value it must be given, not with reference to quantity, but for effect, observing, of course, due precautions to avoid all danger from narcotism. The writer has witnessed the use of the sulphate of morphia in doses of a grain hourly, continued during the twenty-four hours, for several days, in a case of severe epidemic dysentery, without the production of any of the phenomena of narcotism. This case is cited, not as affording any criterion of the quantity of opium to be generally given in cases of dysentery, but as showing the remarkable extent to which the system may be rendered tolerant of the remedy by this disease.

Finally, the use of supporting measures of treatment in this, as in many other diseases, follows as a necessary result of present views as to the tendencies of diseases and the objects of treatment. Dysentery, like most inflammatory affections, is rarely cut short. It must have its course, and if it destroy life, the mode of dying is by asthenia. It follows that so soon as danger to life is threatened, it becomes the great object of treatment to support the powers of the system. This is to be done by alcoholic stimulants and concentrated nutriment. The existence of inflammation constitutes no objection to the employment of stimulants whenever there is danger of death by asthenia, nor to their employment to an extent proportionable to the amount of danger. This is a principle in therapeutics of incalculable importance, which is yet to produce its full influence on medical practice. Concentrated nourishment, consisting of the essence of meat, with milk, and a small proportion of farinaceous food, is an essential part of the supporting treatment. In dysentery, it is important that the diet should consist of principles as purely nutritious as possible, in order to have as little fæcal residue as possible to pass into the large intestine.

Chronic dysentery is extremely rare in northern and temperate climates, but it is a frequent sequel of the acute disease in tropical regions. After our late war with Mexico the hospitals in the larger cities of the Union were filled with soldiers who had returned with chronic dysentery. The prospect of recovery when the chronic form of the disease becomes established, is very small. Sooner or later, it proves fatal, usually after a protracted duration, the patient dying by slow asthenia. Palliation of symptoms, and prolongation of life, are generally the only objects to be attained by treatment. The measures to be pursued for these objects consist of opiates, astringents, tonics, regulated diet, and hygienic precautions.

In the management of acute dysentery the liability of the disease to eventuate in the chronic form is to be considered. Patients should not be too early discharged; and proper measures of diet and regimen, together with appropriate remedies, should be continued until the medical officer has satisfied himself that the recovery is complete.

CHAPTER XIV.

SCORBUTUS, OR SCURVY.

When men are confined for a length of time on a diet consisting only of salted provisions and breadstuffs, they are apt to become affected with a peculiar disease, which, from a Scandinavian word, is termed scorbutus or scurvy. The disease was formerly endemic in northern Europe, recurring regularly in the latter part of the winter, and in early spring; the increasing use of garden vegetables gradually limited its ravages, and since the general cultivation of the potato it is rarely seen. It was at one time the scourge of the mariner. In 1497 Vasco de Gama, in the voyage in which he discovered the Cape of Good Hope, and opened a new route for the commerce of India, lost one hundred men out of one hundred and sixty by scurvy. In 1600, in the expedition which formed the first step to the gigantic power which England has since acquired in the East Indies, out of four vessels, three lost a fourth part of their crews, before reaching the Cape, and the remainder of the men were so weakened that they were unable to work the vessels. Richly laden galleons engaged in the commerce between Spain and her American colonies, have been met with every spar standing, and every sail set, but with the crew all dead of what was well named the seaman's plague. Even as late as the end of the last century, in 1794, the disease reached such a height in the Channel fleet as to become an object of national concern to the English government.

A distinction was formerly attempted between sea-scurvy and land-scurvy, but the two are identical, depending on the same causes, and showing the same symptoms. Extreme cases of the disease are now rarely met with, yet every year mild but isolated cases are seen among the under fed and badly lodged. The extent to which it has prevailed in our little army is remarkable. In the year 1859, by an order of Secretary Floyd, the troops were debarred the use of pickles, sour-krout, dried fruits, and fresh vegetables; and in consequence scurvy made its appearance among them, in the march from Fort Leavenworth to Salt Lake, a distance of nine hundred miles. It is stated (Medical Statistics of the Army of the United States), that in five years, out of an army of fourteen thousand men, there were 2803 cases of scurvy. The occurrence to such an extent of a disease wholly preventable, is disgraceful to the authorities.

The invasion of scurvy is first shown by a pallid and swollen complexion, by depression of spirits, by a sense of weariness, and by indisposition to bodily or mental exertion. A slight bruise, which in health would produce no effect, now causes a soft, indolent swelling, which gradually disappears. The gums early become swollen and spongy, a livid line shows itself on their borders, and they bleed upon the slightest friction; afterwards irregular, granulated, fungous growths show themselves on their edges, rendering their outlines uneven, and more or less covering the teeth. These fungous growths not only bleed on the slightest touch, but frequently break off. As the disease advances the teeth become loose, and sometimes, without previous decay, fall out. The tongue and lining membrane of the mouth present a striking contrast to the appearance of the gums; they are very pale, smooth, and moist. Though at first the patient's appetite may remain good, the breath early becomes fetid, and exceedingly offensive. Petechiæ, or purple or blackish spots, looking as if the part had been severely bruised, soon make their appearance; most marked and extensive in the lower extremities, probably from the effect of gravitation. They are likewise found on the upper extremities, and the body; but are rarely seen upon the face. From extravasation of blood, the cellular tissue over large spaces, particularly in the lower extremities, becomes firm and apparently consolidated, giving the part a hard, brawn-like feel; from the same cause hard nodules and lumps often are felt deep-seated in the tissues of the extremities. The legs are apt to become œdematous, the swelling, at first confined to the ankles, gradually involving the whole extremities. Pains, increased by the erect posture or by locomotion, occur in the feet, legs, thorax, and back; they are often complained of by the patient as rheumatic, and are sometimes so severe as to cause him to groan incessantly. Often the pain in the thorax is accompanied by a sense of constriction, and is aggravated by coughing. In uncomplicated scurvy the mind remains unaffected to the last, with the exception of the depression of spirits already noticed, and in bad cases a profound indifference as to the result.

As the disease advances the patient becomes weaker, often fainting on the slightest exertion. Hæmorrhages, frequently profuse, occur from the nose, gums, lungs, stomach and intestinal canal, &c. The ecchymotic swellings break, and become the seat of scorbutic ulcers. These have swollen, livid edges; their surface presents a loose, rapidly growing, and bleeding fungus, while they secrete a thin sanies mixed with blood. In such cases old sores long since cicatrized, break out afresh, and even the callus uniting a bone broken many years previous is said to have been absorbed, leaving the limb as if freshly broken! Death finally occurs either from syncope or through gradual exhaustion.

Pathological anatomy throws little light upon the disease. Besides the alterations which have been detailed as symptomatic, the blood is dark-colored, fluid, and dissolved, and according to Becquerel and Rodier, is found to be of low specific gravity, and to be deficient in globules and albumen, the fibrin being unaltered or increased in amount. With this alteration of the blood, the spleen is invariably enlarged, often to several times its volume. The efficient cause which produces scurvy has long been a subject of discussion, and is not yet perhaps accurately determined. From the constancy of its occurrence when men have been for a long time confined to a diet composed principally of salt provisions, it was supposed that there was something noxious in salt, something that acted as a poison, when that substance was for a long time taken in excess. But repeated observation has proved that the protracted use of salt provisions under certain circumstances has no effect in producing scurvy; that drinking salt water during the existence of the disease does not aggravate it, and that it may occur when salt provisions form no part of the diet. It has repeatedly appeared in workhouses and prisons, where salted provisions were either not used at all, or formed a very trifling part of the dietary of the inmates; it has raged in camps where fresh meat was abundant; and it has attacked individuals in private life, confining themselves to a diet of fresh meat, bread, and tea. Dr. Christison, who, in the Edinburgh Monthly Journal, has given an interesting record of the disease as it showed itself in the neighborhood of Edinburgh, ascribes its appearance there to a deficiency in the proteinaceous or nitrogenous compounds in the food. He found that in the prison in Perth where scurvy appeared among the prisoners, it showed itself some time after an allowance of treacle had been substituted for the milk previously served out to the prisoners; and that the disease was rapidly cured by an allowance of milk, assisted in some cases by the addition of fresh meat to the dietary of the patient. Analogous facts have been elsewhere reported. But, on the other hand, the dietary of seamen who at present are the principal sufferers from scurvy, is by no means deficient in proteinaceous substances; both albumen and fibrin are abundant in it. Again, often men have been compelled to subsist for a length of time on an allowance of food insufficient for full and perfect nutrition, and though they have become feebler and thinner, scurvy has not been induced. The poor in Ireland and Germany are habitually so circumstanced, but they only become affected with it under peculiar and exceptional circumstances.

One thing is marked in the dietary of those who become affected with scurvy—the complete absence from it of all fresh, esculent vegetables, or their use in exceedingly small quantities. However poor and insufficient a diet may be, so long as it contains potatoes, cabbage, lettuce, onions, or similar vegetables, or so long as it includes a moderate quantity of fresh fruit, whatever other inconveniences or diseases it may occasion, it does not cause scurvy. When scurvy in late years has appeared in alms-houses, prisons, etc., it has appeared in the spring, after a *prolonged* absence from fresh vegetables in sufficient quantity. The effect of lemon-juice in preventing the attack of scurvy was early observed. It was mentioned that in the voyage under Commodore Lancaster to the East Indies in 1600, of four vessels three of them suffered from scurvy to such an extent as to lose one fourth of their crews, and to disable the remainder. On the fourth vessel, commanded by the Commodore himself, every morning three table-spoonfuls of fresh lemon-juice were served out to each of the men, and none of them suffered from scurvy. Yet this fact was entirely lost sight of, and the disease continued to decimate the navy until, in 1795, through the exertions of Dr. Lind and Sir Gilbert Blane, the general use of lemon-juice was introduced among seamen.

The juice of many of the fruits which have proved most efficacious as anti-scorbutics, as that of the orange, lemon, crab-apple, etc., is decidedly acid, and it was supposed that the virtues of the fruit resided in the acid principle; but it was soon found that citric acid was very inferior to lemon-juice as an anti-scorbutic, and that vinegar, acetic and tartaric acids, have no influence whatever. Dr. George Budd suggests that fruit and vegetables act by furnishing to the system some of the organic salts which abound in vegetables, and which are necessary to perfect nutrition. Dr. Garrod proceeds a step further, and maintains that potash is the base of the salt thus furnished. When fresh beef is covered with dry salt, the salt rapidly becomes moist, attracting the juices from the beef, and thus condensing and hardening it. These juices consist of water holding a number of salts in solution, and into these salts potash largely enters. Salted provisions induce scurvy, not from the salt which has been added to them, but from a staminal principle which is abstracted. Again, potash in large proportion is one of the constituents of all fresh vegetables. Cabbage, celery, lettuce, potatoes, scurvy grass, contain it in large quantity. Lime, lemon, and orange juice, contain nearly a grain of potash to every ounce of juice. It has long been remarked that vegetables eaten raw are more efficacious as anti-scorbutics than when cooked. Now one effect of boiling vegetables is the loss of a certain amount of the potash, which remains dissolved in the water. Dr. Garrod quotes from the *Provincial Med. and Surg. Jour.* the dietary of a union workhouse, under which the inmates remained free from anything like scurvy; in this four and a half pounds of potatoes were allowed weekly to each person. On account of the scarcity and high price of potatoes, the same weight of boiled rice was substituted. In a few months the inmates became scorbutic. Now the main difference between rice and potatoes is in the respective amounts of potash which they contain. An ounce of rice yields but .005 of a grain of potash; an ounce of potato a grain and a half. So in the instance quoted by Dr. Christison where treacle was substituted for milk—milk contains potash, which is absent in treacle.

There are a number of circumstances by which the tendency to scurvy or its progress is affected, which have no direct connexion with diet. It occurs most readily in the young, who have not yet completed their growth, and in the aged, in whom all the functions of the body are carried on with less vigor; in the one case the processes of waste and nutrition are both more active, in the other the function of assimilation suffers equally with the remainder of the system. On shipboard it shows itself first among the inactive and indolent, or among those who are subject to too strenuous and long continued exertion. Depression of spirits, foul air, a damp atmosphere, deprivation of solar light, depressing causes acting either upon body or mind, facilitate its invasion and assist its progress. Where from the inadequacy of any of the staminal principles of a diet, the system is trembling on the verge of disease, anything which may impair either digestion or assimilation, or which may promote the waste of tissues, may precipitate the patient into positive illness.

The treatment of scurvy consists in the use of articles which should be given to prevent it: fresh vegetables, ripe fruits, lettuce, cabbage, raw scraped potatoes, &c., or when these cannot be obtained, sour-krout, dried fruits, and desiccated vegetables.

Lemon or orange juice is often the most convenient anti-scorbutic, as it is also the most powerful. An astringent and stimulating gargle may be employed for the mouth, and a bitter infusion administered. When the symptoms of scurvy are subdued, iron may often be given with advantage.

NOTE.—In addition to the remedies mentioned by Dr. McCready, and the value of which has been fully established, we will mention a few others whose reputation is perhaps less known, but which may occasionally be found serviceable.

Assistant-Surgeon A. T. Ridgely reported in 1856, from the cantonment of the Sixth Infantry, Nebraska Territory, the appearance of scurvy among the troops, but it was promptly arrested by the bulb of the wild artichoke, of which the men ate freely.—*Statis. Rep. to Med. Bureau*, 1860, p. 36. Surgeon Madison, stationed at Fort Randall, Mo., speaks also of the wild artichoke as a "most excellent anti-scorbutic." It was found to be edible from the first of April to the middle of May.—*Statis. Rep.*, 1860, p. 40. Surgeon Madison speaks favorably of the wild onion and wild nettles. He adds, moreover, "The Indians eat nothing save fresh game or dried buffalo meat, and they put up for winter quantities of dried plums, buffalo berries, choke berries, &c., hence their immunity."

In a paper published in the *New York Jour. of Med.*, September, 1851, G. Perin, Assistant-Surgeon United States Army, writing from Fort McIntosh, Laredo, Texas, first introduced to the notice of the profession the Agave Americana, or Maguey, a species of cactus, as an anti-scorbutic. It is the same plant from which the drink called "pulque" is manufactured, and is indigenous to Texas, California, and

Mexico. As a remedy for scurvy, Dr. Perin places it far above lime-juice, or any other remedy known to him. Surgeons Johns, Myer, and many others, confirm these statements. It is prepared as follows: the leaves being cut off close to the root, are placed in hot ashes until thoroughly cooked, when they are removed, and the juice expressed from them and strained. It may be given in doses of from two to three ounces three times daily. The internal or white portion of the stalk of the plant is also a wholesome and nutritious food.

Benjamin F. Bache, of the United States Navy, and Director of the Naval Laboratory, Brooklyn, N. Y., informs me that he has used with excellent effect, Turner's old remedy, namely—

Potassæ Nitratis ʒ ij.
Acidi Acetici f. ℥ viij.
M. ft. Sol.
Dose: f. ℥ ss. ter in die.

Citric acid he thinks worthless, and lemon acid not much better; even fresh lemons will sometimes fail to arrest it, but they are better than lemon acid.

Dr. Thomas Turner, Passed Assistant-Surgeon in the Naval Laboratory, has seen old sailors cut potatoes into slices, and then pack them in a barrel with molasses. The molasses preserves the potatoes, and the sailors eat them raw.

APPENDIX.

NOTE A.

This probe is constructed with a notch or slit in one end, for the purpose of conveying tents into wounds.

The accompanying woodcut represents the common bullet forceps, omitted in the text.

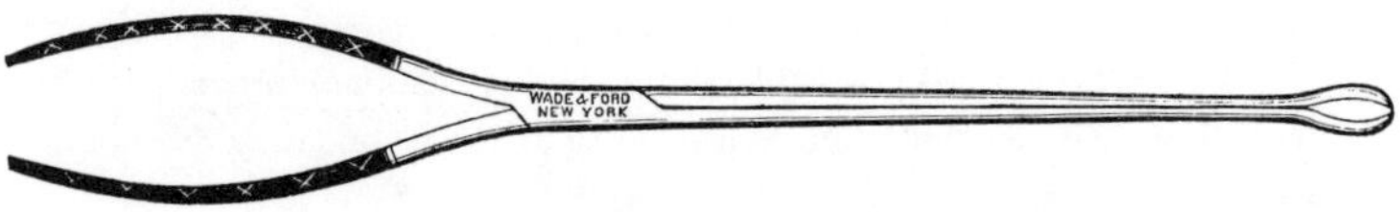

NOTE B.

The first woodcut represents the field tourniquet used in the Prussian service, without a pad; and in which the strap, after passing around the limb, is simply laid over and caught upon the steel points of the buckle. Tourniquets of this construction are sometimes distributed among the soldiers before an engagement.

The second represents the field tourniquet with a pad, and with the strap passing *through* the buckle in the usual manner.

The third represents the same tourniquet slightly modified.

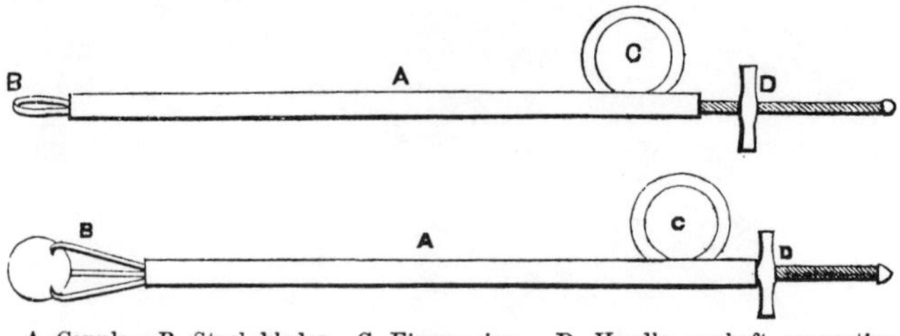

A, Canula. B, Steel blades. C, Finger ring. D, Handle or shaft supporting the blades.

BULLET FORCEPS. Invented by Isaac Moses, M.D., U. S. A.

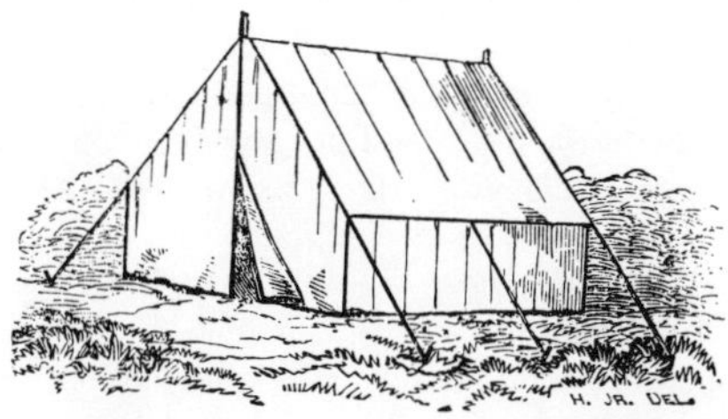

COMMON WALL TENT, OR MARQUEE,

Recommended by United States Army Medical Board, for Hospital purposes.

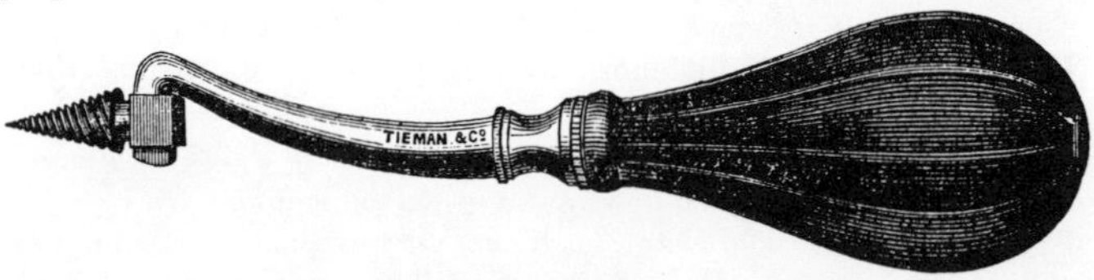

SCREW ELEVATOR.

Found in the author's "Field Case," and intended to screw into the hole made by the pin of the trephine for the purpose of lifting the disk of bone. The screw is movable, and, when taken off, the hook can be used also as a levator.

CAMP AND HOSPITAL COOKERY.

How to soak and plain-boil the Rations of Salt Beef and Pork, on Land or at Sea.—To each pound of meat allow about a pint of water. Do not have the pieces above three or four pounds in weight. Let it soak for seven or eight hours, or all night if possible. Wash each piece well with your hand in order to extract as much salt as possible. It is then ready for cooking. If less time be allowed, cut the pieces smaller and proceed the same, or parboil the meat for twenty minutes in the above quantity of water, which throw off and add fresh. Meat may be soaked in sea water, but by all means boiled in fresh when possible.

It is advisable, at sea, to have a perforated iron box made, large enough to contain half a ton or more of meat, which box will ascend and descend by pulleys; have also a frame made on which the box might rest when lowered overboard, the meat being placed outside the ship on a level with the water, the night before using; the water beating against the meat through the perforations will extract all the salt. Meat may be soaked in sea water, but by all means washed.—*Soyer.*

Meat Soup for twenty-five men.—Meat, twenty-five pounds; water, fifteen quarts; salt, one large tablespoonful; pepper, one teaspoonful; rice, two pounds, put in while boiling; with such fresh vegetables or preserved, as can be obtained—say three pounds.

Pork Soup for twenty-five men.—Pork, twelve pounds; cold water, six gallons; beans, three quarts; rice, two pounds; season; boil one hour and a half, soak the beans over night.

Irish Stew for twenty-five men.—Mutton, veal, beef, venison, or pork, twenty-five pounds; cut into pieces six inches square; onions, four pounds; Irish potatoes, eight pounds; salt, four tablespoonfuls; pepper, one tablespoonful: water, eight quarts. Cook from one to two hours slowly; thicken the gravy with flour mixed into a smooth paste, with water or potatoes, mashed fine.—*Soyer.*

Boiled Meats.—In *boiling* meats it is important to keep the water constantly boiling, otherwise the meat will soak up the water.

If it is necessary to add more water, be careful that it be *boiling* water.

Be careful to remove the *scum*, especially when it first begins to boil, and a little salt thrown in aids in raising the scum.

Put salt meat into cold water, let it heat very gradually forty minutes or so. Fresh meat must be put into boiling water. Allow about *twenty minutes* for boiling for each pound of fresh meat, and *twenty-four* for salt meats.

Do not let the meat remain long after it is done, as it injures it. Put a plate in the bottom to prevent the part that touches from cooking too much.

Be sure not to let the fire get hot, so as to make a hard boiling, especially at first. The more gently meat boils the more tender it is, and the more perfectly the savory portion is developed and retained. If the meat is fat, skim it and save the fat for other purposes.

Put salt into the water about in the proportion of a great spoonful to a gallon.

Salt Pork with Potatoes and Cabbage for twenty-five men.—Pork, fifteen pounds, extract the bones; potatoes, three pounds; two winter cabbages; water, ten quarts; boil for two hours. Serve the meat with vegetables. A good broth may be made from the gravy by adding peas, beans, or rice, and a little onion. Ship biscuit broken into the broth makes an excellent soup.

To Fry Meat.—Heat the frying-pan very hot, put in a little fat pork, then the meat you wish to fry. Season with salt and pepper. When done take out the meat and add a pint of water to the fat in the frying-pan, a few slices of onions, or two teaspoonfuls of vinegar, or a few chopped pickles, or other sauce; thicken with a little flour, and pour it over the cooked meat.

Baking and Roasting with the Field Stove.—By the removal of the caldron, and the application of a false bottom put over the fire, bread bakes extremely well, as well as meat, potatoes, puddings, &c. Bread might be baked in oven at every available opportunity, at a trifling cost of fuel.

Baking in fixed Oven.—In barracks, or large institutions, where an oven is handy, a long iron trough shall be made, four feet in length, with a two story movable grating in it, the meat on the top of the upper one, giving a nice elevation to get the heat from the roof, and the potatoes on the grating under, and a Yorkshire pudding, at the bottom. Four or five pieces of meat may be done on one trough. If no pudding is made, add a quart more water.—*Soyer.*

Chowder.—The best fish for chowder are haddock and striped bass. Cut the fish in pieces of an inch thick, and two inches square. Take six or eight good-sized slices of salt pork, and put in the bottom of an iron pot, and fry them in the pot till crisped. Take out the pork, leaving the fat. Chop the pork fine. Put in the pot a layer of fish, a layer of split crackers, some of the chopped pork, black and red pepper, and chopped onion, then another layer of fish, split crackers, and seasoning. This do till you have used your fish. Then just cover the fish with water, and stew slowly till the fish is perfectly tender. Take out the fish, and put it in the dish in which you mean to serve it; set it to keep warm. Thicken the gravy with pounded cracker; add, if you like, mushroom catsup and Port wine. Boil the gravy up once, and pour over the fish; squeeze in the juice of a lemon, and garnish with slices of lemon.

If not salt enough from the pork, more must be added.

Portable Soup.—Boil down the meat to a thick jelly, season it highly with salt, spices, and wine, or brandy; when cold, cut it in square inches, and dry them in the sun. Keep them in a tight tin vessel, and when you use them put a quart of boiling water to one or two of the cakes, which should be one inch square, and the fourth of an inch thick. Vegetables can be added.

Tea for twenty-five men.—Water, twelve quarts; twelve teaspoonfuls tea; inclose the tea in a cloth tied up very loosely, and throw it into the boiler while it is boiling hard; let it remain for a moment, then take off the boiler, cover it, and let it stand ten minutes, when it will be ready for use.—*Soyer.*

Coffee for twenty-five men.—Water, twelve quarts; when it boils add twenty ounces of coffee; mix well, and leave it on the fire until it boils again; take it off, and pour in a little more than a quart of cold water; let it stand in a warm place ten minutes, when it will be settled. Now decant into another vessel, leaving the dregs in the first.—*Soyer.*

Baked Beans.—Pick over the beans the night before, and put them in warm water to soak, where they will be kept warm all night. Next morning pour off the water, and pour on boiling water, and let them stand and simmer till the beans are soft, and putting in with them a nice piece ot pork, the skin gashed. Put them into the deep dish in which they are to bake, having water just enough to cover them. Bury the pork in the middle, so that the top will be even with the surface. All the garden beans are better for baking than the common field bean. They must bake in a moderately hot oven from two to three hours.

Common Mode of Cooking Rice.—To a pint of clean rice, put three quarts of cold water and a teaspoonful of salt. Boil it fifteen or twenty minutes, then pour off the water, add milk and some cream, and let it boil a few minutes longer. It should not be so soft as to lose its form.

In case you wish to fry it next morning, boil it longer in the water, and omit the milk, or not, as you please.

Home-brewed Yeast.—Boil a handful of hops half an hour in three pints of water. Pour half of it, *boiling hot*, through a sieve, on to nine spoonfuls of flour, mix, and then add the rest of the hop water. Add a spoonful of salt, half a cup of molasses, and *when blood warm*, a cup of yeast.

Wheat Bread of Home-brewed Yeast.—Sift eight quarts of flour into the kneading tray, make a deep hole in the middle, pour into it a pint of yeast, mixed with a pint of lukewarm water, and then work up this with the surrounding flour till it makes a thick batter. Then scatter a handful of flour over this batter, lay a warm cloth over the whole, and set it in a warm place. This is called sponge.

When the sponge is risen so as to make cracks in the flour over it (which will be in from three to five hours), then scatter over it two tablespoonfuls of salt, and put in about two quarts of wetting, warm, but not hot enough to scald the yeast, and sufficient to wet it. Be careful not to put in too much of the wetting at once.

Knead the whole thoroughly for as much as half an hour, then form it into a round mass, scatter a little flour over it, cover it, and set it to rise in a warm place. It usually will take about one quart of wetting to four quarts of flour.

In winter, it is best to put the bread in sponge over night, when it must be kept warm all night. In summer, it can be put in sponge early in the morning, for if made over night it would become sour.

Brown Bread.—One quart of rye; two quarts of Indian meal; if fresh and sweet, do not scald it; if not, scald it; half a teacup of molasses; two teaspoonfuls of salt; one teaspoonful of saleratus; a teacup of home-brewed yeast, or half as much distillery yeast. Make it as stiff as can be stirred with a spoon with warm water. Let it rise from night till morning. Then put it in a large deep pan, and smoothe the top with the hand dipped in cold water, and let it stand a while. Bake five or six hours. If put in late in the day, let it remain all night in the oven.

Kentucky Corn Dodgers.—Three pints of *unsifted yellow* corn meal; one teaspoonful (heaped) of lard; one pint of milk; work it well, and bake in cakes the size of the hand, and an inch thick.

Baked Indian Pudding.—Three pints of milk; ten heaping tablespoonfuls of Indian meal; three gills of molasses; a piece of butter, as large as a hen's egg. Scald the meal with the milk, and stir in the butter and molasses, and bake four or five hours. Some add a little chopped suet in place of the butter.

Milk Porridge.—Make a thin batter with Indian meal and wheat flour, a spoonful of each, and pour it into a quart of boiling milk and water, equal portions of each. Salt it to the taste. Boil ten minutes.

Water Gruel.—To two quarts of boiling water add one gill of Indian meal and a heaped tablespoonful of flour, made into a paste and stirred in the water. Let it boil slowly twenty minutes. Salt, sugar, and nutmeg to the taste.

Oatmeal makes a fine gruel in the same way.

Beef Tea.—Broil a pound of tender, juicy beef ten minutes, salt and pepper it, cut in small pieces, pour on a pint of boiling water, steep it half an hour, and then pour it off to drink.

Arrowroot and Tapioca Gruels.—Jamaica arrowroot is the best. Make a thin paste, and pour into boiling water, and flavor with sugar, salt, and nutmeg. A little lemon juice improves it.

Tapioca must be soaked in twice the quantity of water over night, then add milk and water, and boil it till it is soft. Flavor as above.

Simple Wine Whey.—Mix equal quantities of water, milk, and white wine. Warm the milk and water, and then add the wine. Sweeten it to the taste.

Essence of Beef.—Tender and juicy beef is cut into small pieces, and then put into a strong stone bottle, corked tightly, and placed in a kettle of cold water; the water is to be heated until it boils. Let it boil an hour, then pour off, strain and season.

Milk Punch.—Brandy, one ounce; cold milk, half a pint; sweeten, and add a little grated nutmeg.

INFORMATION FOR PERSONS DESIROUS OF ENTERING THE MEDICAL STAFF OF THE U. S. ARMY.

No person can receive the appointment of Assistant Surgeon in the army of the United States, unless he shall have been examined and approved by an Army Medical Board, to consist of not less than three Surgeons or Assistant Surgeons, to be designated for that purpose by the Secretary of War; nor can any person receive the appointment of Surgeon in the army of the United States, unless he shall have served five years as an Assistant Surgeon, and unless, also, he shall have been examined by an Army Medical Board, constituted as aforesaid.

Boards of Medical Examiners are convened at such times as the wants of the service render it necessary, when selections are made by the Secretary of War of the number of applicants to be examined for appointment of Assistant Surgeon. To the persons thus selected, invitations are given to present themselves to the Board for examination. These invitations state the time and place of meeting of the Board.

Applicants must be between twenty-one and thirty years of age. The Board will scrutinize rigidly the moral habits, professional acquirements, and physical qualifications of the candidates, and report favorably in no case admitting of a reasonable doubt.

The Board will report the respective merits of the candidates in the several branches of the examination, and their relative merit from the whole; agreeably whereto, if vacancies happen within two years thereafter, they will receive appointments and take rank in the Medical Corps.

An applicant failing at one examination may be allowed a second, after two years; but never a third.

Applications must be addressed to the Secretary of War; must state the residence of the applicant, and the date and place of his birth. They must also be accompanied (*references will receive no attention*) by respectable testimonials of his possessing the moral and physical qualifications requisite for filling creditably the responsible station, and for performing ably the arduous and active duties of an officer of the Medical Staff.

No allowance is made for the expenses of persons undergoing these examinations, as they are indispensable pre-requisites to appointment; but those who are approved and receive appointments will be entitled to transportation on obeying their first order.

The pay and emoluments of Surgeons and Assistant Surgeons are shown by the following table:

	Pay per month.	No. of rations per day.	Amount of rations per month.	No. of horses for which forage is alowed.	Amount for forage per month.	Servants.						Aggregate amount receivable.
						No. for which pay is allowed.	Amount allowed for pay per month.	Amount allowed for clothing per month.	Amount allowed for rations per month.	Total amount allowed per month.		
Assistant Surgeon, under five years' service . .	$53 33	4	$36	1	$8	1	$12	$2 50	$9	$23 50		$120 83
Assistant Surgeon, over five years' service . .	70 00	4	36	1	8	1	12	2 50	9	23 50		187 50
Assistant Surgeon, over ten years' service . .	70 00	8	72	1	8	1	12	2 50	9	23 50		173 50
Surgeon, under ten years' service	80 00	4	36	3	24	2	24	5 00	18	47 00		187 00
Surgeon, over ten years' service	80 00	8	72	3	24	2	24	5 00	18	47 00		223 00

The allowance for forage and servants is only paid to the Surgeons and Assistant Surgeons when they actually employ and keep in service the number of servants and horses charged for.

In addition to the above, Surgeons and Assistant Surgeons are allowed an additional ration per day, after the termination of every five years' service.

War Department, *January*, 1860.

The Board mentioned in the accompanying advertisement is now in Session at the Metropolitan Hotel, N. Y.

War Department, Adjutant General's Office.
Washington, March 13, 1861.

Special Orders, No. 76.

A Board of Medical Officers will assemble in New York city on the 1st day of May next, or as soon thereafter as practicable, for the examination of Assistant Surgeons for promotion, and of such candidates for appointment as may be invited to present themselves before the Board.

DETAIL FOR THE BOARD.

Surgeon Clement A. Finley,
" Charles McDougall,
" W. J. Sloan.

By order of the Secretary of War:

L. THOMAS, Adjutant-General.

INFORMATION FOR PERSONS DESIROUS OF ENTERING THE MEDICAL STAFF OF THE U. S. NAVY.

It is prescribed by law that no person shall be appointed in this branch of the service who has not been examined and found qualified by a board of Naval Surgeons, designated by the Secretary of the Navy.

A board of Naval Surgeons will be assembled annually, at such place as may be indicated by the Department, usually about the close of the lecture season of the colleges, for the examination and selection of candidates for admission into the Medical Corps of the Navy, as well as for the examination of Assistant Surgeons who may be candidates for promotion.

Application for permission to attend the examination for admission to the Medical Corps of the Navy must be addressed to the Secretary of the Navy, stating the age and residence of the applicant, and be accompanied by respectable testimonials of his possessing the moral and physical qualifications requisite for filling creditably the responsible position of a Medical Officer of the Navy.

The application of no one will be considered who is under twenty-one or over twenty-five years of age.

The permission will state the time and place of the meeting of the board.

The board rigidly scrutinizes the physical qualifications of each candidate, as well as his moral, mental, and professional fitness for the Naval Service; and reports favorably upon no case admitting of a reasonable doubt, as the health and the lives of the officers and men of the Navy are objects too important to be intrusted to ignorant or incompetent persons.

The board reports the relative merit of the candidates as shown by the examination; and appointments will be made in the Navy as vacancies may occur, in the order in which they may be reported by the board.

No qualified candidate will be held over for appointment beyond one year; if not appointed within that time, it will be necessary for the candidate to be re-examined, when he will take position with the class last examined.

Physical examination will precede the professional; no candidate, not physically qualified for the active duties of the service, will be examined professionally. The board will make a separate report in each case, of the physical condition, *direct* to the Department, to be placed on file with the testimonials of the candidate.

No allowance is made for the expenses of persons undergoing these examinations, as they are indispensable prerequisites to appointment.

After five years' service in the Navy, at least two years of which shall have been passed "on board a public vessel of the United States at sea," Assistant Surgeons shall be entitled to an examination for promotion.

In order that the relative position of Assistant Surgeons of the same date, who shall be examined for promotion at different times, may be more readily determined, a majority of the members of the board will be selected, if practicable, from those who served on the next preceding board.

Assistant Surgeons, who are candidates for promotion, shall present to the board testimonials of correct deportment and habits of industry from the Surgeons with whom they have been associated on duty; also, a journal of Practice, or Case-Book, in their own hand-writing. They are expected to be familiar with all the details of duty specified in the "Instructions for the Government of Medical Officers."

Any Assistant Surgeon who shall fail to present himself for examination after he has been ordered (unless for reasons which may be satisfactory to the Department), or who, after examination, shall be reported by the board as "not qualified" for promotion, shall be dropped from the list of Officers of the Navy.

ISAAC TOUCEY, *Secretary of the Navy.*

COMPENSATION.

The pay of Assistant Surgeons and Surgeons is established by act of Congress, approved on the 1st June, 1860, and is as follows:

SURGEONS.

Every surgeon on duty, at sea, for the first five years after the date of his commission as surgeon, two thousand two hundred dollars.

For the second five years after the date of his commission as surgeon, two thousand four hundred dollars.

For the third five years after the date of his commission as surgeon, two thousand six hundred dollars.

For the fourth five years after the date of his commission as surgeon, two thousand eight hundred dollars.

For twenty years and upwards after the date of his commission as surgeon, three thousand dollars.

Fleet surgeons, three thousand three hundred dollars.

Every surgeon on other duty, for the first five years after the date of his commission as surgeon, two thousand dollars.

For the second five years after the date of his commission as surgeon, two thousand two hundred dollars.

For the third five years after the date of his commission as surgeon, two thousand four hundred dollars.

For the fourth five years after the date of his commission as surgeon, two thousand six hundred dollars.

For twenty years after the date of his commission as surgeon, two thousand eight hundred dollars.

Every surgeon on leave or waiting orders, for the first five years after the date of his commission as surgeon, one thousand six hundred dollars.

For the second five years after the date of his commission as surgeon, one thousand eight hundred dollars.

For the third five years after the date of his commission as surgeon, one thousand nine hundred dollars.

For the fourth five years after the date of his commission as surgeon, two thousand one hundred dollars.

For twenty years and upwards after the date of his commission as surgeon, two thousand three hundred dollars.

PASSED ASSISTANT SURGEONS.

Every passed assistant surgeon on duty at sea, one thousand five hundred dollars.

When on other duty, one thousand four hundred dollars.

When on leave or waiting orders, eleven hundred dollars.

ASSISTANT SURGEONS.

Every assistant surgeon on duty at sea, one thousand two hundred and fifty dollars.

When on other duty, one thousand and fifty dollars.

When on leave or waiting orders, eight hundred dollars.

NAVY DEPARTMENT, *Jan.* 2, 1861.

The Board of Naval Surgeons will convene at the Brooklyn Naval Hospital for the examination of candidates, on the 1st day of June, 1861. There are thirty-nine vacancies to be filled.

No more medical gentlemen are wanted at present to supply *temporarily* the places of surgeons on board of the transports. Surgeons who have entered in this way are not in the line of promotion.

INFORMATION FOR WOMEN DESIROUS OF ACTING AS ARMY NURSES.

WOMEN'S CENTRAL RELIEF ASSOCIATION,
Cooper Union, Room No. 25, 1st Floor.

The Ladies and Societies who have undertaken the preparation of the necessary supplies for the relief of the Soldiers of our Army, on the field or in the hospitals, are respectfully informed that the Women's Central Relief Association, which proposes to combine the efforts of such Societies, has opened an office at Room No. 25 of the Cooper Union. The office will be open daily, from 10 o'clock A.M. to 2 o'clock P.M.

Models and patterns of all articles mentioned in the appended list will be kept on exhibition, for examination and reference, at the office, and all necessary instructions will be given for their preparation by an authorized person. Patterns will also be sent by mail to those desiring them and sending six postage stamps. All contributions of articles mentioned in the following list will be received at the office of the Association, between the hours of 9 o'clock A.M. and 4 o'clock P.M., by our authorized agent, Mr. George Roberts, and a receipt given for the same.

Public acknowledgment through the papers will be made weekly, by the Board of Managers, of all contributions and donations.

All contributions of Clothing, Lint, Bandages, Bedding, &c., will be immediately forwarded to the depot, at the Spingler Institute, while all comforts in the way of eatable stores will be retained and distributed on requisition from the Medical Purveyor of the Army.

DR. W. H. DRAPER,
MRS. FITZGERALD,
MRS. T. D'OREMIEULX,
MRS. G. L. SCHUYLER,
Sub-Committee of the Executive Com.
VALENTINE MOTT, M.D., *President.*
GEO. F. ALLEN, *Secretary.*

LIST OF HOSPITAL AND FIELD SUPPLIES FOR THE SICK AND WOUNDED, SUGGESTED BY THE RELIEF ASSOCIATION.

1. Bandages—For assortment and proportionate numbers of each variety required, see Regimental Supply for three months.
2. Lint—Scraped and ravelled in equal proportions, packed in boxes of uniform size.
3. Old Linen and Cotton Cloth, without selvage or seams, for compresses.
4. Ring Pads and Cushions.
5. Cotton Batting and Cotton Wadding; fine Flax and Sponges.
6. Red Flannel, in the piece.
7. Bookbinders' Board, for Splints; pieces 18 inches by 4 inches.
8. Saddlers' Silk for Ligatures, Skeins waxed and wound on cards.
9. Sewing Needles, assorted, in cases; Linen, Thread, Tape, and Scissors.
10. Adhesive Plaster, Camel-Hair Pencils, Oiled Silk, Oiled Muslin, India Rubber and Gutta Percha Cloths, in the piece.
11. Wrapping Paper.
12. Cotton Bed Shirts—1½ yards long, 2 breadths of unbleached muslin 1 yard wide, open one-half yard at the bottom, length of

Sleeve three-quarters yard, length of Arm Hole 12 inches, length of Collar 20 inches, length of Slit in front 1 yard, fastened with four tapes.

Loose Muslin Drawers—1¼ yards long with a breadth of 1 yard wide muslin in each leg, with a hem and drawing string round the waist and the bottom of each leg; length from waist to crotch on the back 22 inches, and in the front 18 inches, with 3 buttons and button-holes.

Short Bed Gowns—made like long, only 1 yard long, and open in front.

13. Dressing Gowns of double calico, of which a paper pattern can be furnished.
14. Bed Sackings of ticking, 1 yard wide and 2 yards long.
15. Muslin sheets, 4 feet wide and 8 feet long.
16. Pillow Sacks of ticking, 16 inches wide and 30 inches long. Pillow-Cases of muslin, one-half yard wide, 1 yard long.
17. Towels.
18. Eye-Shades of green silk, with elastics.

Various articles have been named in the newspapers as desirable gifts for the use of the sick and wounded. The following are added as of especial value: Juice of beef, as stock for beef tea, put up in sealed cans; arrowroot, packed in light wooden boxes of one pound each; brandy; white wine, for wine whey, etc.; champagne in small bottles, for cases of sudden sinking; china feeders of different sizes for administering nourishment where the head cannot be moved; bent glass tubes for similar use; castile soap for washing wounds; old table linen to serve as soft towels; distilled vinegar; cans of fruit; whiskey; tobacco; handkerchiefs, slippers, socks; crackers or biscuits; sub-acid fruit; tea, sugar, cocoa; pure lemon syrup; oatmeal.

REPORT OF THE REGISTRATION COMMITTEE ON THE SELECTION AND PREPARATION OF NURSES FOR THE ARMY.

ADOPTED BY THE BOARD OF MANAGERS.

As there exists at present in the public mind very little positive knowledge in relation to army nursing, it is of great importance that certain facts should be widely circulated, which will show to all, and particularly to the women interested in this subject, what can and what cannot be accomplished by them. It is believed that when the conditions under which army nursing by women is alone possible and proper are fully understood, much of the noble enthusiasm of women, whose sole desire is to serve their country in this momentous crisis, will be directed into other channels, where intelligent and patriotic effort is imperatively called for.

The first fact to be distinctly understood is this, viz. that women have not hitherto been employed in military hospitals as nurses. The nursing is done by soldiers drafted out of the ranks for that purpose, and there is no provision whatever for boarding, paying, or in any way recognising women in the capacity of nurses to sick soldiers. Women, therefore, who now go on to Washington with the idea of nursing, go there on their own responsibility, and find themselves without recognition by the authorities, with no proper provision for their support, and with no work to do. There is now a considerable number of these volunteer nurses in Washington. A letter has already been received by a member of our board from Miss D. L. Dix, containing an informal request from the authorities that no more volunteer lady nurses be encouraged to come on *until officially requested*, as it would prove embarrassing to have more there at present.

At the same time, we have received from the Chief Medical Bureaux of the Army the following statement, to wit: that the plans now in progress under the direction of this Association, and the hospitals of this city, receive the full approbation of the proper authorities, and that the services of the bands of nurses selected and proposed under those plans will be gratefully accepted whenever such services can be consistently called into requisition.

The second fact to be widely known is this, viz. that nursing in military hospitals is a very different thing from nursing in civil hospitals, and still more from private nursing. The class of patients to be nursed, the character of the under nurses, who will always be men, the social isolation of the position, and the absolute necessity of enforcing military discipline, combine to render nursing in military hospitals a service of peculiar difficulty, which can only be accomplished successfully by a select and disciplined band of nurses. Of course, such service could not be rendered by the young and inexperienced, nor by those possessing delicate constitutions, nor by persons of unsteady character. Women in middle life, intelligent, trustworthy, and zealous in their work, are the suitable individuals from whom this band should be formed.

In accordance with the above views, and guided by the printed records of Miss Nightingale's invaluable experience in army nursing, and the testimony of military surgeons, the following regulations for selecting candidates have been drawn up—these regulations being approved by the Hospital Association, to whom they were submitted:

Age.—Each candidate must be between the ages of thirty and forty-five, exceptions being only made in the case of nurses of valuable experience.

Health.—Only women of strong constitutions will be received; chronic disease, or other physical weakness, disqualifying for service.

Character.—Every applicant must present a written testimonial or introduction from a responsible person who can be seen. If the applicant be accepted, these testimonials will be filed, and the name of the referee entered on the register of nurses. Only persons of the highest respectability will be received. While the utmost delicacy is used in such investigation, the requisition of morality, sobriety, honesty, and trustworthiness will be rigidly enforced.

Discipline.—A promise of cordial compliance with all the regulations of the service will be required; the subordination of nurses to the general superintendent, and of all to the medical authorities, being distinctly insisted on. Each candidate will be required to sign the printed regulations of the service.

Dress.—A regulation dress will be appointed by the board, which each nurse will be required to adopt, no hoops being allowed in the service. A committee on outfit will be appointed to superintend the wardrobe of the nursing corps, which will be regulated by the amount of baggage allowed to each individual.

Admission.—Each registered candidate will receive a ticket of admission signed by the Secretary of this Board. She will take this ticket to the Hospital Committee for counter-signature, and will then enter upon the course of instruction arranged by Physicians and this Board.

Number of Candidates.—The number of names required will necessarily be limited, for each woman must be qualified to act as a chief or head nurse. Ten Bands, or a class of one hundred, will now be enrolled, due notice being given in the daily journals when the lists are full. Should a second corps be needed, the call will again be published in the papers.

REGULATIONS FOR THE MEDICAL DEPARTMENT OF THE UNITED STATES ARMY.

PUBLISHED BY ORDER OF THE PRESIDENT OF THE UNITED STATES,

March 6, 1860.

"Nothing contrary to the tenor of these present regulations will be enjoined or allowed in any part of the forces of the United States, by any commander whatever."

The senior medical officer of a hospital will distribute the patients, according to convenience and the nature of their complaints, into wards or divisions, under the particular charge of the several assistant surgeons; and will visit them himself each day as frequently as the state of the sick may require, accompanied by the assistant, steward, and nurse.

His prescriptions of medicine and diet are written down at once in the proper register, with the name of the patient and the number of his bed; the assistants fill up the diet table for the day, and direct the administration of the prescribed medicines. He will detail an assistant surgeon to remain at the hospital day and night, when the state of the sick requires it.

In distributing the duties of his assistants, he will ordinarily require the aid of one in the care and preparation of the hospital reports, registers and records, the rolls, and descriptive lists; and of another in the charge of the dispensary, instruments, medicines, hospital expenditures, and the preparation of the requisitions and annual returns.

He will enforce the proper hospital regulations to promote health and prevent contagion, by ventilated and not crowded rooms, scrupulous cleanliness, frequent changes of bedding, linen, &c.

He will require the steward to take due care of the hospital stores and supplies; to enter in a book daily, the issues to the wardmasters, cooks, and nurses; to prepare the provision returns, and receive and distribute rations.

He will require the wardmaster to take charge of the effects of the patients; to register them in a book, to have them numbered and labelled with the patient's name, rank, and company; to receive from the steward the furniture, bedding, cooking utensils, &c., for use, and keep a record of them, and how distributed to the wards and kitchens; and once a week to take an inventory of the articles in use, and report to him any loss or damage to them, and to return to the steward such as are not required for use.

The cooks and nurses are under the orders of the steward; he is responsible for the cleanliness of the wards and kitchens, patients and attendants, and all articles in use. He will ascertain who are present at sunrise, and sunset, and tattoo, and report absentees.

At surgeon's call the sick then in the companies will be conducted to the hospital by the first sergeants, who will each hand to the surgeon, in his company book, a list of all the sick of the company, on which the surgeon shall state who are to remain or go into hospital; who are to return to quarters as sick or convalescent; what duties the convalescents in quarters are capable of; what cases are feigned; and any other information in regard to the sick of the company he may have to communicate to the company commander.

Soldiers in hospital, patients or attendants, except stewards, shall be mustered on the rolls of their company, if it be present at the post.

When a soldier in hospital is detached from his company so as not to be mustered with it for pay, his company commander shall certify and send to the hospital his descriptive list and account of pay and clothing, containing all necessary information relating to his accounts with the United States, on which the surgeon shall enter all payments, stoppages, and issues of clothing to him in hospital. When he leaves the hospital, the medical officer shall certify and remit his descriptive list, showing the state of his accounts. If he is discharged from the service in hospital, the surgeon shall make out his final statements for pay and clothing. If he dies in hospital, the surgeon shall take charge of the effects, and make the reports required in the general regulations concerning soldiers who die absent from their companies.

Patients in hospital are, if possible, to leave their arms and accoutrements with their companies, and in no case to take ammunition into the hospital.

When a patient is transferred from one hospital to another, the medical officer shall send with him an account of his case, and the treatment.

The regulations for the service of hospitals apply, as far as practicable, to the medical service in the field.

The senior medical officer of each hospital, post, regiment, or detachment, will keep the following records, and deliver them to his successor: a register of patients, a prescription book, a diet book, a case book, a meteorological register, copies of his requisitions, annual returns, and reports of sick and wounded; and an order and letter book, in which will be transcribed all orders and letters relating to his duties.

He will make the muster and pay rolls of the hospital steward and matrons, and of all soldiers in hospital, sick or on duty, detached from their companies, on the forms furnished from the Adjutant General's office, and according to the directions expressed on them.

The extra pay allowed to soldiers acting as cooks and nurses in hospitals will be paid by the Pay Department. Such extra services will be noted on the extra muster rolls, and for the sums thus expended the Pay Department will be reimbursed by the Medical Department.

He will select the cooks, nurses, and matrons, with the approval of the commanding officer. Cooks and nurses will be taken from the privates, and will be exempt from other duty, but shall attend the parades for muster and weekly inspections of their companies at the post, unless specially excused by the commanding officer.

Ordinarily, hospital attendants are allowed as follows: to a general hospital, one steward, one nurse as wardmaster, one nurse to ten patients, one matron to twenty, and one cook to thirty; to a hospital where the command exceeds five companies, one steward and wardmaster, one cook, two matrons, and four nurses; to a post or garrison of one company, one steward and wardmaster, one nurse, one cook, and one matron; and for every two companies more, one nurse; at arsenals where the number of enlisted men is not less than fourteen, one matron is allowed. The allowance of hospital attendants for a regiment in the field will be, for one company, one steward, one nurse, and one cook; for each additional company, one nurse; and for commands of over five companies, one additional cook.

Medical officers where on duty will attend the officers and enlisted men, and the servants and laundresses allowed by law; and, at stations where other medical attendance cannot be procured, and on marches, the hired men of the army, and the families of officers and soldiers. Medicines will be dispensed to the families of officers and soldiers, and to all persons entitled to medical attendance; hospital stores to enlisted men.

Medical officers, in giving certificates of disability, are to take particular care in all cases that have not been under their charge, and especially in epilepsy, convulsions, chronic rheumatism, derangement of the urinary organs, ophthalmia, ulcers, or any obscure disease liable to be feigned or purposely produced; and in no case shall such certificate be given until after sufficient time and examination to detect any attempt at deception.

A board of not less than three medical officers will be appointed from time to time by the Secretary of War, to examine applicants for appointment of assistant surgeons, and assistant surgeons for promotion. And no one shall be so appointed or promoted until so examined and found qualified.

The board will scrutinize rigidly the moral habits, professional acquirements, and physical qualifications of the candidates, and report favorably, either for appointment or promotion, in no case admitting of a reasonable doubt.

The Secretary of War will designate the applicants to be examined for appointment of assistant surgeon. They must be between twenty-one and twenty-five years of age. The board will report their respective merits in the several branches of the examination, and their relative merit from the whole; agreeably whereto, if vacancies happen within two years thereafter, they will receive appointments and take rank in the medical corps.

When an assistant surgeon has served five years, he is subject to be examined for promotion. If he decline the examination, or be found not qualified by moral habits or professional acquirements, he ceases to be a medical officer of the army.

An applicant for appointment failing at one examination, may be allowed a second after two years; but never a third.

The Secretary of War will appoint from the enlisted men of the army, or cause to be enlisted, as many competent hospital stewards as the service may require, not to exceed one for each post.

The senior medical officer of a hospital requiring a steward may recommend a competent non-commissioned officer or soldier to be appointed, which recommendation the commanding officer shall forward to the Adjutant General of the army, with his remarks thereon, and with the remarks of the company commander.

The commanding officer may re-enlist a hospital steward at the expiration of his term of service, on the recommendation of the medical officer.

As the object of the act of August 16, 1856, in holding out the inducement of a more permanent appointment, was to procure the services of a more competent body of hospital stewards, no soldier, nor citizen, must henceforth be recommended for appointment under that act who is not *known* to be temperate, honest, and in every way reliable, as well as sufficiently intelligent, and skilled in pharmacy, for the proper discharge of the responsible duties likely to be devolved upon him.

The following Rules are from the General Regulations of the U. S. Army :—

Before the action, the quartermaster of the division makes all the necessary arrangements for the transportation of the wounded. He establishes the ambulance depots in the rear, and gives his assistants the necessary instruction for the service of the ambulance wagons, and other means of removing the wounded.

The ambulance depot to which the wounded are carried or directed for immediate treatment, is generally established at the most convenient building nearest the field of battle. A red flag marks its place, or the way to it, to the conductors of the ambulances, and to the wounded who can walk.

The active ambulances follow the troops engaged, to succor the wounded and remove them to the depots. For this purpose, the conductors should always have the necessary assistants, that the soldiers may have no reason to leave the ranks for that purpose.

The medical director of the division, after consultation with the quartermaster general, distributes the medical officers and hospital attendants at his disposal, to the depots and active ambulances. He will send officers and attendants, when practicable, to the active ambulances, to relieve the wounded who require treatment before being removed from the ground. He will see that the depots and ambulances are provided with the necessary apparatus, medicines, and stores. He will take post and render his professional services at the principal depot.

If the enemy endanger the depot, the quartermaster takes the orders of the general to remove it or to strengthen its guard.

The wounded in the depots, and the sick, are removed, as soon as possible, to the hospitals that have been established by the quartermaster-general of the army, on the flank or rear of the army.

THE END.

INDEX.

DERROM'S HUTS AND COTTAGES.

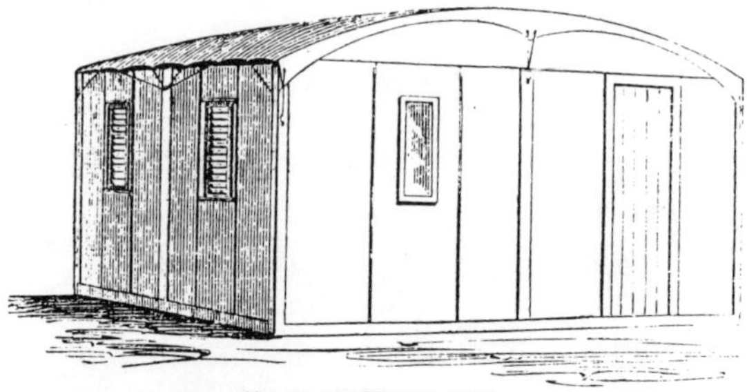

PLAIN MILITARY HUT.

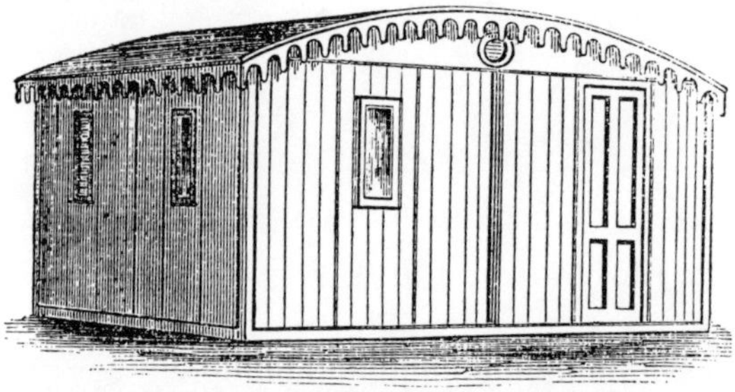

FOR OFFICERS.

Can be used for permanent or other Camps; for Hospital purposes; for temporary Dwellings in Town, in the Country, or at Sea Side; for Railroad or other Contractors, &c., &c.

Can be put up or taken down in a few minutes.

A NEW PORTABLE HUT.—The Hut is twelve feet square, and can be put together in ten minutes. It is believed to be superior to tents, in that it is dry, has a floor, will not wear out or blow down, gives good ventilation, and a man can stand in any portion of it. Although for convenience it is better to have but one size, yet any number of them can be connected so that a company, or a regiment, can be housed together if desirable. For hospitals, or permanent camps, it is decidedly superior to tents, and the ease with which it is put together suggests its use wherever a camp can be approached by steamers, railroads, or wagons.

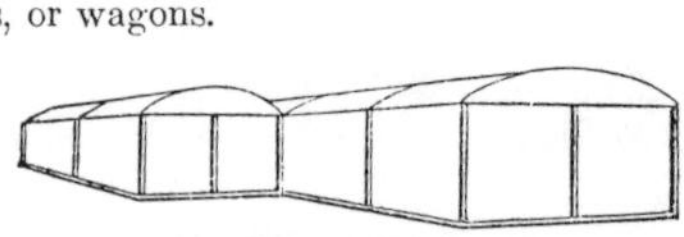

COMBINATION.

Parties wishing these Huts for private use, can have any amount of additional ornaments added to the doors, windows, &c., to suit any taste. For light or ventilation the windows or rolling blinds can be placed in any position or shape—square, oval, circular, gothic, &c., &c.

The proprietor has an extensive STEAM CARPENTRY in Paterson, N. J., where orders for the above can be filled at the shortest notice.

For information address A. DERROM, PATERSON, N. J.
Refers to H. V. BUTLER & CO., 13 PARK PLACE, N. Y.

FRASER. A Treatise on penetrating wounds of the Chest. 8vo. London, 1859. $1 55.

GILL. An Epitome of Surgery. 32mo. London, 1860. 30c.

GOFFRES. Precis Iconographique des bandages, pansements, et appareils. In 12mo., avec planches coloriées. Paris, 1858. $9 50.

GROSS, (S. D.) A Manual of Military Surgery; or, Hints on the Emergencies of Field, Camp, and Hospital Practice. 24mo. Philadelphia, 1861. 50c.

GUTHRIE, (G. J.) Commentaries on the Surgery of the War in Spain, Portugal, France, and the Netherlands; with Additions relating to those in the Crimea in 1854-55. Revised to October, 1855. 6th edit. crown 8vo. London, 1855. $4 65.

HAMILTON, (F. H.) A Practical Treatise on Fractures and Dislocations. 8vo. Philadelphia, 1860. $4 25.

HENNEN. Principles of Military Surgery. 8vo. London. (Scarce.) $5 50.

JACQUOT. Du Typhus de l'Armée d'Orient. 8vo. Paris, 1838. $1 75.

LARREY. Clinique chirurgicale exercée particulierement dans les camps et les Hopitaux Militaires depuis 1792 jusqu'en 1836. Paris, 1830–1836, 5 forts vols. in-8, atlas de 47 pl. $10 00.

LARREY. Memoires de Chirurgie Militaire. 4 vol. 8vo. Paris, 1812. $7 00.

LYONS. A Treatise on Fever, or Selections from a Course of Lectures on Fever. 8vo. London. 1860. $3 87.

MACLEOD, (G. H. B.) Notes on the Surgery of the Crimean War; with Remarks on Gunshot Wounds. London. $3 37.

MAILLOT ET PUEL. Aide Memoire Medico-Legal de l'Officier de Santé de l'Armée de Terre; ouvrage dans lequel sont traitées toutes les questions de droit relatives à la Medicine Militaire, à l'operation medicale du Recrutement, etc. Publié par l'autorité du Ministre de la Guerre. 8vo. Paris, 1842. $1 87.

MARROIN. Histoire Medicale de la flotte Francaise, dans la Mer Noire, pendant la guerre de Crimée. 8vo. Paris, 1861. $1 00.

MASSY. On the Examination of Recruits, intended for the use of young Medical Officers on entering the Army. London. $1 55.

MEDICAL STATISTICS of the U. S. Army, from 1819 to 1860. 1 vol. 8vo., and 2 vols 4to. $14 00.

MEYNNE. Hygiene Militaire. Etudes sur la construction des Casernes, sur l'alimentation du Soldat, et sur les fatigues de la vie Militaire. 8vo. Bruxelles, 1856. $1.25.

NELATON. Elemens de Pathologie Chirurgicale. 5 vols. 8vo. Paris, 1844 to 1859. $9.50.

PLAIES D'ARMES A FEU, des Communications faites à l'Academie Nationale de Medecine par Baudens, Roux, Malgaigne, Amussat, Velpeau, Bessin, &c. 8vo. Paris, 1849. $1.00.

RECUEIL de Memoires de Medicine, Chirurgie et Pharmacie Militaires publié par ordre du Ministre de Guerre. 1st Serie 1816 à 1846. 61 vols. 8vo.
2d Serie, 22 vols. each $1.75.
3d Serie, 1860, " 1.75.

RECORDS OF DAILY PRACTICE: A Scientific Visiting List for Physicians and Surgeons.

CONTENTS:

Present State of Patients	72 double pages.
Microscopical Examinations	4 pages.
Obstetrical Engagements	4 "
Vaccination "	4 "
Consultation and other Professional Engagements	4 "
List of Nurses and Address	2 "
Meteorological Observations and Endemic Influences	4 "
Miscellaneous Memoranda	6 "
Index of Patients	4 "

This little book is not intended to supersede the use of a regular visiting list; its aim, as the title indicates, is to supply a medium for taking notes of the state of the patient, as soon after the visit as it is possible, and whilst the facts are still fresh in the memory. In hospital practice, we believe it will be found invaluable. The arrangement, under the head of "*Present state of the patient,*" is admitted, by competent judges, to be all that could be desired.

Price in cloth 50 cents, or in pocket-form, 75 cents, by mail, free on the receipt of the price.

SAUREL. Memoire sur les Fractures des Membres par Armes à feu. 8vo. Montpellier, 1856. 75 cents.

SCRIVE. Relation Medico-Chirurgicale de la campagne d'Orient. 8vo. Paris, 1857. $2.00.

STROMEYER. Fractures of Limbs occurring in Gunshot Injuries. 8vo. London. $1.55.

TRIPLER & BLACKMAN. A Handbook for the Military Surgeon, being a compendium of the duties of the Medical Officer in the Field. 12mo. Cincinnati. 1861. $1.00.

VALLEIX. Guide du Medecin Praticien, ou Resumé General de Pathologie Interne et de Therapeutique Appliquée. Quatrieme Edition, Revue, Augmentée, et contenant le resumé des travaux les plus recents, par MM. les Docteurs V. A. Racle et P. Lorain. 5 vols. Grand in 8vo. de chacun 900 pp. Paris. $11.70.

WILLIAMSON, (G.) Notes on the wounded from the mutiny in India, etc. 8vo. Illustrated by 10 plates. London, 1859. $3.25.

Norman Publishing is a division of Jeremy Norman & Company, Inc., leading international dealers in rare books and manuscripts in the history of medicine and science.

The following people collaborated on the production of *A Practical Treatise on Military Surgery:*

Diana Hook, Associate Editor
Steven Hiatt, Copy Editor
Jill Rotenberg, Project Manager
Martha Steele, Editorial Assistant
Seventeenth Street Studios, Designer

The layout was done by Donna Kelley at Zetatype Desktop Publishers of San Francisco, using Ventura Publisher. The type is Bodoni, a Postscript font from Adobe Systems.

Linotronic output by Pinnacle Type, San Francisco.

Printed and bound by Braun-Brumfield, Inc., Ann Arbor.

With its geometrical framework, the Norman Publishing logo resembles the constructed letters of the Renaissance, but there the resemblance ends. The logo incorporates the capital letter N within an arc of the logarithmic spiral, one of the most beautiful mathematical curves appearing in nature. It links together the graphic arts and the sciences, reflecting the dual commitments of Norman Publishing.

NORMAN
PUBLISHING TM